MODELS FOR MENTAL DISORDER

FIFTH EDITION

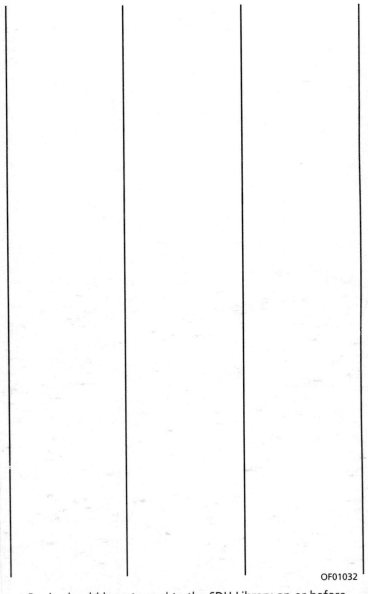

MODELS FOR MENTAL DISORDER

Conceptual Models in Psychiatry

FIFTH EDITION

Peter Tyrer
MD FRCP FRCPsych FFPHM FMedSci
Professor of Community Psychiatry, Centre for Mental
Health, Department of Medicine,
Imperial College, London, UK

With Illustrations by Derek Steinberg

WILEY Blackwell

This edition first published 2013 © 2013 by John Wiley & Sons, Ltd
Previous editions © 1987, 1993, 1998, 2005 by John Wiley & Sons, Ltd

Registered Office
John Wiley & Sons, Ltd, The Atrium, Southern Gate, Chichester, West Sussex, PO19 8SQ, UK

Editorial Offices
9600 Garsington Road, Oxford, OX4 2DQ, UK
111 River Street, Hoboken, NJ 07030-5774, USA

For details of our global editorial offices, for customer services and for information about how
to apply for permission to reuse the copyright material in this book please see our website at
www.wiley.com/wiley-blackwell

Library of Congress Cataloging-in-Publication Data

Tyrer, Peter J., author.
  Models for mental disorder : conceptual models in psychiatry / Peter Tyrer. – Fifth edition.
    p. ; cm.
  Includes bibliographical references and index.
  ISBN 978-1-118-54052-7 (pbk.)
  I. Title.
  [DNLM: 1. Mental Disorders. 2. Models, Biological. 3. Models, Psychological. WM 140]
  RC437.5
  616.89–dc23

                              2013017990

A catalogue record for this book is available from the British Library.

Wiley also publishes its books in a variety of electronic formats. Some content that appears in print may not
be available in electronic books.

Cover image: © Derek Steinberg

Set in 10/12pt Palatino by SPi Publisher Services, Pondicherry, India
Printed and bound in Malaysia by Vivar Printing Sdn Bhd

1   2013

CONTENTS

Preface vii

Acknowledgements ix

1   Introduction 1

2   The Disease Model 9

3   The Psychodynamic Model 41

4   The Cognitive-Behavioural Model 69

5   The Social Model 103

6   An Integrated Model 123

Appendix: Teaching Exercise 179

Glossary of Terms 181

Index 187

PREFACE

A great deal has happened to mental health in the 26 years since the first edition of this book was published. Rather shamefacedly in retrospect, we intended it originally to be a guide for psychiatrists and students in the mental health professions only when we first conceived the book. At that time the people who received mental health care and their relatives had only distant knowledge of how psychiatrists viewed their world. Now everything is different and I would like to think this is for the better. Mental health professionals can no longer hide behind jargon, obfuscation, half-truths and their perceived status in their interactions with others. Their activities are now centre stage and open to scrutiny from their other colleagues, regulatory bodies, patient lobby groups of various sorts, professionals from other disciplines, and the general public. 'What are you doing, what is the reasoning behind it, and what is the likely outcome?' are the questions everybody is asking. Of course, this is not only true of mental health professionals but indeed of all medical practitioners in this new spirit of openness. The problem mental health professionals have is they are not singing from the same hymn book; the cacophony of sound emanating from their vocal chords is not harmonious or synchronized. The aim of this book is to explain why, but not to criticise unduly, and instead to attempt a synchronization that makes the mental health choir a joy to listen to.

To do this I have brought up to date each of the four major models of mental disorder and added extra interlocking pieces that make the integrated model a more successful one. Because I understand that many who receive psychiatric services are naturally keen to know more about the reasoning behind their care, the language has been edited slightly to make it more readable and easily understood. But I apologise if I have failed in my task here. For the past 10 years I have been editor of the *British Journal of Psychiatry* and have tried to improve the readability of the journal while maintaining high scientific standards. The sad fact is that high scientific standards usually go with very turgid reading and I hope that I have been able to overcome this to some extent.

You will note that the pronoun 'we' has now become 'I' in this fifth edition. I am very sad to report that my fellow author and illustrator, Derek Steinberg, died shortly after the last edition of this book in 2006, but I have retained most of his cartoons as they remain a fitting memory for his talents. Derek was more of an adherent to the psychodynamic model than the others in this book and I do hope in editing this particular chapter I am being fair to his aims and intentions. We had great fun in piecing together the different chapters of this book and throughout this time, despite many arguments, I never once heard Derek raise his voice. This is not easy when negotiating with an irascible academic with strong feelings and in the editing of this fifth edition I have imagined Derek sitting behind me and reminding me that I need to tone down some of my more extreme views. I would like to think that he has succeeded here but that is for the reader to decide.

I should like to thank my editorial colleagues in the Royal College of Psychiatrists, particularly those who had been serving on the Janitor Committee, for helping me to maintain my precarious position on a rickety fence separating the domains of the adherents of each of my four models, when judging papers for publication. They have helped me to agree that all models can win and all can have prizes. I also thank Peter Lee, a model social worker, and my wife, Helen, for helping me to develop the social model much more coherently, and for the development of nidotherapy, which owes a great deal, much more than she may realize, to her. Finally, I must acknowledge the contribution of my twin cats, Running Thunder and Chasing Small, for being secure custodians of my manuscript, and for acting as my flanking cavalry as we move into the jousting arena where the battle of the models will begin.

ACKNOWLEDGEMENTS

This fifth edition has been helped greatly by the discussions I have had with many outside the field of psychiatry. These particularly include my wife, Helen, whose experience in general medicine, general practice and cognitive-behavioural therapy has helped enormously in my understanding of how we are seen by others, and also by colleagues in general medicine where we have recently been involved in many studies in liaison psychiatry. I have also had many stimulating and amusing arguments with Sandra O'Sullivan and Clinical Studies Officers in the North London hub of the Mental Health Research Network that have also altered my views, I hope for the better. When you are involved with trying to persuade patients to take part in research studies in mental health you realize that both they and their carers, including other physicians, have widely disparate views about mental health and the many models that underlie interventions. These have convinced me that models of mental disorder will continue to be constructed, sometimes crazily, often inappropriately, but always with some value, for many years to come, and, despite all their failings, we would be lost without them.

1

INTRODUCTION

Welcome to models for mental disorder. It may seem an odd subject, but it is not peripheral to understanding of mental illness. Many years ago I was responsible for the undergraduate teaching programme in psychiatry at our medical school. One of our students showed great aptitude in the subject and told me that he would like to specialize in psychiatry after he qualified. I gave him every encouragement, not least as this subject tends to be low on medical student career priorities. I did not think much more about it until I saw him shortly after his final examinations, where he achieved distinction in psychiatry, but also in some other subjects too. He was looking a little discomfited when I saw him and I asked him if anything was the matter. He told me he had just come out from a two-hour meeting with the Dean of the medical school. He added at some length exactly what had happened. 'I have heard a rumour that you want to specialize in psychiatry,' said the Dean, 'this can't be correct, can it?' The student said it was. 'What on earth do you think you are doing?' said the Dean. 'Psychiatry is not a proper part of medicine. People tend to go into it if they fail at everything else, but you are an outstanding student who ought to be doing something better.' 'I've considered all the options, sir,' said the student, 'but I feel more comfortable with specializing in mental health than any other part of medicine and I feel I can be of more value there.' 'But psychiatry is not a scientific subject,' expostulated the Dean, 'it has no proper base. Most of the people practising it rely on their experience and opinion only. Do you really want to specialize in a subject where everyone has different views and it is the loudest voice that wins, not science?'

The conversation went on in this way for some time and what really surprised the student was how much prejudice there seemed to be against the subject of psychiatry. The interview was entirely counter-productive; the student was

Models for Mental Disorder: Conceptual Models in Psychiatry, Fifth Edition. Peter Tyrer.
© 2013 John Wiley & Sons, Ltd. Published 2013 by John Wiley & Sons, Ltd.

even more determined to specialize in mental health after it took place and subsequently enjoyed an extremely successful career in the subject, never doubting that this was the right choice of career. But although this account could just be cited as yet another example of stigma and prejudice against mental health, it is also possible to look further and understand why other doctors look at psychiatry askance, and why from a distance it appears to be a subject with no clear philosophy, rhyme or reason. Doctors in general medicine, if asked what model they practise, would probably ask the questioner to repeat the question, as it is not one which they would normally think about. They practise the disease model, the one described in the first chapter in this book, and because they have been taught right from the beginning of their training in this model, they recognize it as the truth rather than a model, as they could not contemplate looking at the subject in any other way. Psychiatry has tried hard to adopt the disease model but despite valiant efforts to make it work, it only covers part of psychiatry. John Bucknill, the founding editor of the journal I currently edit, the *British Journal of Psychiatry*, stated right from the beginning of his editorship that insanity was a disease of the brain (Bucknill, 1856), and as this hypothesis was first expressed by Hippocrates it cannot be ignored. The way psychiatry has developed in the past 150 years has shown that a simple disease model is not adequate to explain everything we know about mental health and illness, and at various times other models have entered the fray.

We all like to have a coherent basis for our actions; professionals in mental health, and this includes many disciplines – psychiatrists, psychologists, mental health nurses, occupational therapists, social workers, and care workers of all types – are no exception in wishing to have a clear underpinning philosophy behind what we do. Most of these practitioners, usually implicitly, adopt one of the models discussed in the following pages. Explicitly they may claim that they come to a considered judgement on each clinical issue and adopt the appropriate model for that judgement. This is commonly described as being 'eclectic'. Now eclectic means 'deriving ideas from different sources' and although it sounds impressive it describes neither a model nor a philosophy. In practice there is a danger that the eclectic follows admitted or undeclared prejudices without realizing what these are. It allows a luxury of change without necessarily giving a reason for this and is not far short of dilettantism, the adoption of different models almost as a whim.

Models cause psychiatrists endless trouble and none of the models of mental illness described in this is so neat and elegant that it covers everything. Each of them conveniently leaves out the rough pieces that do not fit and the search is still on for a model that is truly comprehensive and can be applied universally. The Dean who interviewed our medical student almost certainly belonged to the group who consider psychiatry to be a 'soft' branch of medicine in which the theoretical framework for treatment is poor, there are too many disparate treatments, and there is much argument between practitioners, and this probably explains the fundamental prejudice towards psychiatry that still lies behind the subject in medicine (Bolton, 2012), and which is shared by the general population. We have just completed a study of a common condition, health anxiety, in medical patients attending five different types of clinic in general hospitals. We saw nearly 30,000 patients and 5747 (19%) of these had abnormal health anxiety (that is, it created considerable concern, worry and handicap) (Tyrer *et al.*, 2011). We offered those who had high levels of health anxiety the opportunity of taking part in a randomized trial of a new psychological treatment for this condition. Fewer than one in 12 (444) of these, agreed to take part or were excluded for other reasons. I would like the reader to hazard a guess how many of 5747 patients suffering from cancer, or indeed Alzheimer's disease, would respond if asked to take part in a trial of a new treatment for their condition. Whatever your guess, I am sure it would be much higher than 8%. The reasons people gave for not taking part in our trial included a mix of denial (there is nothing wrong with me that the proper doctors cannot sort out), shame (I do not need any special help and should be able to sort this out on my own), fear (I don't trust these newfangled psychological treatments), and prejudice (I won't have anything to do with mental health services). My view is that stigma, discrimination and ignorance of mental health by many outside the subject is related to the models that are discussed in this book. Unfortunately, some of this prejudice is related to the oldest model of all, that mental illness is a form of degeneracy, a rotting of the brain that has no cure, only primitive forms of alleviation. This was the view of mental illness by many so-called experts in the nineteenth century which has unfortunately persisted, particularly in less-developed communities, to the present day, and which explains why in many low-income countries mental health receives less than 1% of the total health budget.

In each of Chapters 2–5 one of the models is described in its most favourable light. Chapter 2 chapter will look at mental disorders in which the cause, clinical manifestations, pathology and treatment of many organic illnesses seem now to be very well known and so are admirably suited to the disease model. Unfortunately, as we shall find, the disease model creates tremendous antipathy among many other mental health professionals who have been trained in different ways and seems to have no bearing on their practice. They are using one or more different models, each of them creating some antipathy in others, and if they are not exposed and compared, there will be confusion and continued argument, and our medical school Dean will have more justification for his arguments.

So rather than present a cosmetic repair of the schisms in psychiatric thought, in this book we are exposing these divisions from the beginning. In the following chapters we leave each model to speak for itself in explaining the cause, pathology and treatment of a number of mental disorders and show how each is interpreted using the model under consideration. An adversarial approach is used here. Each model is presented to its best advantage and the other models criticized for their less satisfactory positions. We recognize this may make each model a little two-dimensional and look like a caricature of the real thing. However, we hope that by exposing the conflict between different models the reason for their relative persistence becomes clear and there is much greater understanding between those who hold to one model at the expense of others. It should also help the reader to understand the philosophy of those who particularly adhere to one model or another and find that it suits most of their needs. It also prepares the reader for the integrated model in the final chapter. We do not pretend that the synthesis here is going to satisfy everybody but at least it offers a framework for use in practice, and I feel after 40 years of practice that it is the best working model available, even though, as you will read, it still creates controversy. The very fact that so many models for mental disorder still exist shows that there is a place for all of them. But in time a unified approach will have to come.

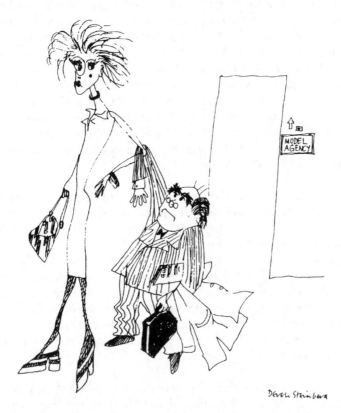

'Models cause psychiatrists endless trouble . . .'

What is described here is hardly new. Siegler and Osmond in 1974 described six different models: medical, moral, psychoanalytic, family, conspiratorial and social, and came down very heavily in favour of the medical model. We have confined our attention to four: the disease, psychodynamic, cognitive-behavioural and social models. The reason why we have done this is that in clinical practice each of the models goes about treatment in a different way and therefore shows the differences between each model in ordinary practice. You will note that we have not used the term 'medical model'. We agree with Bursten (1979) that this adjective is a confusing and unnecessary one. It gives more attention to the practitioner (a doctor) than this description, and because it does not actually describe the type of model, it can be manipulated to suit any taste. However, we accept that some people might regard the final synthesis that we present later in this book as a true medical model and this is fairly close to what has been called the bio-psychosocial model following the pioneering suggestions of George Engel over 35 years ago (Engel, 1977).

This is not intended to be a short textbook of psychiatry but could be seen as a philosophical introduction around the subject. We are dealing here with ideas, views and opinions, and these are no substitute for the bricks and mortar of hard fact. However, each model has to be tested in the factual world and we expose each one to scrutiny in this way. Our main aim is the practical one of making sense of the presentation in mental illness. At its simplest level we are trying to teach a sorting operation, rather like the tests often given to young children, when they are required to separate a number of articles on the basis of shape, size or colour. If this book serves its purpose it should be possible to identify each new piece of psychiatric information and place it with the appropriate model. There should be little difficulty in identifying the right model for a particular description or interpretation, although this is sometimes hard to decipher in the use of psychiatric jargon. So Lady Macbeth's question 'cans't thou not minister to a mind diseased, pluck from the heart a rooted sorrow?' can be seen easily as a question from the psychodynamic model, even though Shakespeare had no idea what this model was – although some say he was the first psychoanalyst. The idea that a deeply rooted mental problem can cause current distress is one of the fundamental tenets of the psychodynamic model and it is clear that Lady Macbeth is looking for such an answer in asking her question. This view receives confirmation later in the play when she declares 'throw physic to the dogs, I'll none of it'. This clear rejection of the disease model in favour of the psychodynamic one is entirely consistent.

Similarly, when Hamlet says, 'how strange or odd soe'er I bear myself, as I perchance hereafter shall think meet, to put an antic disposition on', he is following the ideas behind the social model. He is trying to find a solution to the mad incestuous relationships going on in his family but it is not he who is mad, but the Danish court environment in Elsinore.

Of course this sorting process is only the first stage in using models properly. The hackneyed phrase 'I can see where you are coming from' describes the recognition and identification of the model being used. Once we identify the correct model, instead of a pot-pourri of isolated facts and opinions, we can understand the coherence and the belief systems that lie behind statements, opinions and the interpretation of events and symptoms in mental disorder. Because treatment is so closely linked to each model the disturbingly large range of therapies competing with each other in psychiatry also comes into perspective. In guiding the practitioner and patient to a synthesis of these models we recognize that each individual has to make a personal synthesis. This is an exercise that demands a great deal but may well repay amply in the long term. We are not expecting every reader to get to the stage of making a personal model of mental disorder but at least those views that are already held will be recognized as components of a model rather than nuggets of truth. Both an honest self-assessment and understanding of the various ways in which psychiatry is practised are the first steps in getting to grips with the subject. We hope it will develop a common language of understanding so that mental health workers can understand each other, students and aspiring clinicians can understand them, and patients, clients or users (however we wish to describe them according to which model we use) can understand what on earth is going on when they puzzle about the motives and actions of their therapists.

Since the first edition of this book in 1987 users of mental health services have gained enormously in power. Recently I became aware of this when I complained to the hospital management that one of the patients on the ward I was looking after was creating many problems for other patients and really should be moved elsewhere. My request was ignored but when I suggested to the most vulnerable patient concerned that she made the request it was acted on immediately. 'Doctor knows best' has not yet been replaced with 'patient knows best' but there is now much greater awareness of the need to involve patients (I'm sorry I still find it very difficult to use the term 'service users' as the alternative here) in our decisions and the reasons for them. One of the commonest phrases in clinical research is 'informed consent'. This describes the understanding of the subject that what is being carried out is fully appreciated and agreed to by them and signed accordingly. Mental health workers are much better practitioners if they also have informed consent from the subjects that they treat. This is not a restricted exercise in which only a small part of the reasons for treatment are shared. Ideally it should explain the models being used so that the patient can act with reciprocity, the real underpinning of properly informed consent. Listening to the patient is the first part of model development; explaining to the patient using the same model, or contradicting it by introducing another, is a necessary precursor to getting agreement over treatment.

So now we would like the reader to take on the role of spectator observing a play. In each of the next four chapters the actors have different roles. Some may resonate more positively than others but all can be said to be viable. The model army is now on display.

REFERENCES

Bolton, J. (2012) 'We've got another one for you!' Liaison psychiatry's experience of stigma towards patients with mental illness and mental health professionals. *The Psychiatrist*, **36**, 450–454.

Bucknill, J.C. (1856) The diagnosis of insanity. *British Journal of Psychiatry*, **2**, 229–245.

Bursten, B. (1979) Psychiatry and the rhetoric of models. *American Journal of Psychiatry*, **136**, 661–665.

Engel, G.L. (1977) The need for a new medical model: a challenge for medicine. *Science*, **196**, 129–136.

Siegler, N. and Osmond, H. (1974) *Models of Madness: Models of Medicine*. Macmillan, New York.

Tyrer, P., Cooper, S., Crawford, M., *et al.* (2011). Prevalence of health anxiety problems in medical clinics. *Journal of Psychosomatic Research*, **71**, 392–394.

2

THE DISEASE MODEL

'The main claim of the physical approach, that is the assumption that mental disorders are dependent on physiological changes, is that it is a useful working hypothesis. It has made great advances and looks like making more. It is in line with the main front of biological advance. It is here where psychiatry belongs.'

Eliot Slater, 1954 (in Sargant and Slater, 1954)

'I don't operate on the same wavelength as he does. He sees everybody as a walking brain.'

(Community Mental Health Team Social Worker)

How do we reconcile these two extreme views? One, written at a time when psychoanalysis was the main headline grabber in psychiatry, now seems eminently reasonable. Any abnormality of the mind must ultimately have its origin in some malfunction of pathophysiology of the nervous system, and if we were able to elucidate this it would both help our understanding and promote its correction. The second indicates frustration with this approach when it is carried out to what is perceived as an absurd or excessive degree. Does the concentration on pathophysiology prevent understanding of the person? The proponent of the disease model says 'No, this is nonsense. The person coming to see me wants a problem sorted out. It is my job to isolate this problem from the rest of the person and try and solve it, not to take the whole person into the reckoning. This only dilutes the focus of my enquiry and provides nothing of real use'.

Eight years ago there was a policy in the United Kingdom called 'New Ways of Working'. This was an initiative supported by the Royal College of Psychiatrists and the National Institute for Mental Health in England (2005), in which the position of the psychiatrist was downgraded to that of 'team member' only. This of course was described in Orwellian Newspeak as a 'new model of distributed responsibility and leadership', but the message was clear, the special

Models for Mental Disorder: Conceptual Models in Psychiatry, Fifth Edition. Peter Tyrer.
© 2013 John Wiley & Sons, Ltd. Published 2013 by John Wiley & Sons, Ltd.

skills of the psychiatrist, as a doctor specializing in mental disorders, were being downgraded. The diktat was, 'Just as we may need an occupational therapist to advise us on the daily activities of a patient, we may need you as a psychiatrist from time to time to say something about diagnosis'.

Not surprisingly, this message did not go down well with psychiatrists who considered that mental illness was indeed brain disease and needed the special knowledge of people trained in this discipline. So 37 of the psychiatrists got together and wrote a special article which was published in the *British Journal of Psychiatry*. Entitled 'A wake-up call for British psychiatry', it spelt out exactly what should be expected from psychiatrists when they were asked to assess patients. The two paragraphs below summarize the essentials of their argument, and although the writers were not specifically promoting the disease model – as you will note that they were generous in allowing other approaches to be considered – they did put their fingers on the number of the problem. Unless you know about proper disease in the way that other doctors appreciate it, you cannot say that an adequate mental health assessment leading to a coherent treatment plan can be created by another health professional.

'Psychiatry is a medical specialty. We believe that psychiatry should behave like other medical specialties. When a general practitioner is confident that a psychiatric assessment is *not* needed, it should be possible for a referral to be made directly to a relevant non-psychiatric professional. However, where the general practitioner is unclear about diagnosis or treatment, the patient should be assessed by the most appropriately skilled and experienced professional on the team, the psychiatrist. This is analogous to managing back pain, where in many instances a general practitioner is confident that a medical orthopaedic opinion is not needed and will refer directly to a physiotherapist or an alternative therapist such as an osteopath or chiropractor. However, in severe, persistent or otherwise complex cases an orthopaedic referral should be made, because an assessment by an orthopaedic surgeon is required to ensure accurate diagnosis and exclude or treat causes that are remediable, thereby improving the patient's quality of life and minimizing the risk of complications such as paralysis.

In psychiatry, it is psychiatrists, who are trained in diagnosing physical and mental illness, who are competent to formulate diagnoses that incorporate physical, mental and social factors and, where appropriate, recommend initiation of one or more of a range of possible medical treatments. As in other medical specialties, initial assessment may also involve important contributions from other non-medical members of the team, and may include relevant medical investigations such as blood tests or imaging investigations. Assessment, in many cases, may lead the psychiatrist, as a leader in the clinical team, to conclude that the most suitable treatment is a psychological or social intervention delivered by the member of the team with the most appropriate skills. This approach allows the patient the benefit of a thorough, broad-based assessment by a highly trained professional in order that the most appropriate management is implemented at the earliest opportunity'.

(Craddock *et al.*, 2008)

The rest of this chapter puts more flesh on the bones of this argument, and has the merit of being able to draw on over 2000 years of experience with the disease model in medicine.

WHAT IS DISEASE?

The name 'mental illness' implies disease, and wrapping it up in euphemistic terms such as 'mental health problems' is only a temporary disguise. An illness suggests that there is a fundamental impairment of normal function and is not just a normal variation. The disease model regards mental malfunction as a consequence of physical and chemical changes primarily in the brain but sometimes in other parts of the nervous system. It is a model that has served general medicine extremely well over the last millennium and has made dramatic strides in the past 200 years. Unless it is implied that in mental illness there are different rules that apply to the recognition of illness than in other parts of medicine, we have to adopt the same approach. Thus we have to conclude that in all mental illness there is impaired function and some pathological change in one or more parts of the body.

The definition of disease in this context has been defined by Scadding (1967) as 'the sum of the abnormal phenomena displayed by a group of living organisms in association with a specified common characteristic or set of characteristics by which they differ from the norm for their species in such a way as to place them at a biological disadvantage'. This definition is equally suited to physical and mental disease and is important because it sets limits to illness. In psychiatry, for example, there is much concern over the medicalization of illness by the introduction of new conditions such as 'late luteal dysphoric disorder' (pre-menstrual tension to you and me) and 'social anxiety disorder' (a touch of shyness) that are not necessarily biologically disadvantageous and which merge imperceptibly into normal health variation. The disease model in psychiatry helps to decide which of these conditions is beyond its scope and unsuitable for mental health interventions.

STAGES OF IDENTIFICATION OF DISEASE

There are basically four stages of the identification of disease:

1 The description of symptoms and main features of the disorder (the clinical syndrome)
2 Identification of pathology (i.e. the structural or biological changes created by the illness)
3 Study of the course (natural history) of the syndrome
4 Determination of its cause or causes.

FOUR TENETS OF THE DISEASE MODEL
• Mental pathology is always accompanied by physical pathology
• The classification of this pathology allows mental illness to be classified into different disorders which have characteristic common features
• Mental illness is handicapping and biologically disadvantageous
• Cause of mental illness is explicable by its physical consequences

Management or treatment based on the pathology of illness and its outcome following that treatment (prognosis) can also be considered as part of the model. But if every other stage is properly elucidated these will follow automatically. These stages can only be regarded as logical if four tenets of mental illness are accepted (Box 2.1).

STAGE 1 – IDENTIFICATION OF THE CLINICAL SYNDROME

Almost invariably the recognition of a clinical syndrome is the first stage in the identification of an illness. This begins by first noting *'an association of signs and symptoms'* (signs being observed abnormalities or those identified on examination and symptoms being complaints or *felt* changes in function). Thus certain symptoms such as loss of appetite and lack of energy, or objective signs such as a rapid pulse and an enlarged thyroid gland, tend to be linked to certain illnesses. Once the investigator's mind is alerted to this link other symptoms or signs are identified until the complete syndrome is found. The persistent association of two symptoms or signs may be a chance finding, three is likely to imply a real association, and four confirms it. Observation is the hallmark of correct identification of the syndrome and depends on clinical skills alone. The different elements of the syndrome may have no obvious meaning at first but they will all have to be accounted for if a syndrome is to achieve the status of a disease. Doctors such as Sydenham and Bright in the eighteenth century were excellent examples of medical detectives who identified new important syndromes, and unlike modern doctors they did not have the technology of the laboratory to help them in their task. Psychiatry is not that much further on than we were in eighteenth century and many of our 'diseases' are provisional ones in which several current combined diagnoses (often called comorbidity) may need to be joined together when their real nature has been elucidated.

The great fictional detective, Sherlock Holmes, was modelled by Arthur Conan Doyle on the clinical skills of a well-known Scottish physician, Sir Charles Bell, who was famed for his ability to diagnose medical conditions from small tell-tale signs that no-one else had noticed, which he used to display with a flourish when teaching medical students. So 'Elementary, my dear Watson', could well have come directly from one of these dramatic teaching sessions when a hapless student was used as a foil for the great diagnostician.

Through clinical observation (and interrogation) such doctors identified diseases which were only shown to have the other attributes of the disease model many years later. For example, acute Bright's disease is an inflammation of the kidney (nephritis), first described in 1827. Bright suspected that the syndrome of fever, swelling of the face and hands and little or no flow of urine (anuria) was likely to involve the kidney, but until he linked all the clinical symptoms together the illness went unrecognized. It was many years later before the microscopic pathology (an inflammation of certain structures (glomeruli) of the kidney) and the cause (hypersensitivity to certain strains of a bacterium (the haemolytic streptococcus)) were discovered, but it was Bright who first focused the eyes of science on the problem.

Clinical syndromes are later refined into diagnoses, which are really convenient code names for the syndromes. So when doctors talk together about a patient with thyrotoxicosis (Graves' disease) they are telling each other in one word that the patient has a syndrome which is likely to include an enlarged thyroid gland (goitre) together with atypical facial appearance, loss of weight, abnormal trembling, special eye signs, rapid heartbeat, increased speed of reflexes, and nervousness. The diagnosis of an illness may not be confirmed until other tests (usually carried out in a laboratory) are also consistent with the disease in question but the important part of the diagnostic process is the clinical assessment of the patient, and a clinical diagnosis can stand independently of laboratory findings.

The clinical syndrome is elicited mainly from a detailed history from the patient and a careful physical examination. The history gives strong clues about the possible nature of the complaint, so the doctor is sensitized to pay special attention to certain features when he carries out his examination. Because a history can be unreliable or may omit important changes he or she should always carry out a full physical examination; even if an abnormality expected from the history is identified other abnormal signs may be missed unless all systems are examined.

Taking the history

Every medical student learns this basic approach at an early stage in training; it is also expected by the general public. Psychiatrists who follow the disease model have a very similar approach in assessing mental symptoms using the same techniques as with physical ones. The first stage is a careful history which is more detailed and usually takes longer than a medical history. This is because the background of the patient, his personal and family history and antecedent events are assessed as well as any relevant medical and psychiatric history. All psychiatrists, whatever model they adopt, have to take the whole person into account in making an assessment, and because they are often thinking about the complexities of possible syndromes when they are doing their assessments, they may appear to be impersonal and unaware of their potential to induce distress.

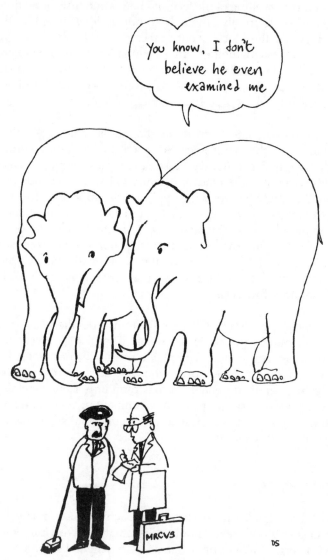

The good clinicians of the past were all too well aware of the importance of good interaction with their patients, but they had the advantage of less knowledge and very little in the way of useful interventions. Indeed, as Dr Jonathan Miller has noted in his television presentations of the history of medicine, before 1900 the practice of medicine involved virtually no effective treatments whatsoever apart from the clever manipulation of placebos (interventions that did no harm but made the person feel better, even if only temporarily).

Although every doctor is now taught diligently about the importance of communication skills it is not always necessary to take on all the tenets of what is commonly called the 'holistic approach' when focused on disease. If you consult a doctor for removal of a wart (verruca) on your finger you might take exception to a set of searching questions about your personal and sexual life on the grounds that this information was irrelevant to wart removal.

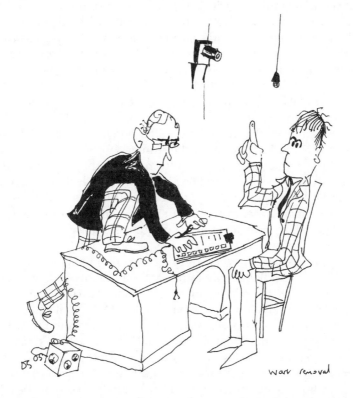

Wart removal

(Of course it might not be irrelevant if the wart was elsewhere.) The psychiatrist who follows the disease model is sometimes criticized for not thinking of the patient as a person, but as a 'case'. The criticism, which is common in other branches of medicine, is only justified if the doctor treats the problem wrongly because of inadequate assessment. The psychiatrist who looks on a mental disorder as a brain disease cannot afford to neglect a full history of past and present problems as this gives important clues to the nature of the disorder. Where he will differ from his colleagues who follow different models is that his questions will be more formalized and the interactional part of the interview ignored. The interview is regarded as an exercise to gain information instead of the first phase in a significant personal relationship.

Examining the patient

The physical examination is carried out in the same way as in other medical conditions, and is an essential part of the assessment of every psychiatric patient, even though it may provide no additional information, as only a few psychiatric disorders have obviously abnormal physical signs. Some psychiatrists disregard a physical examination on the grounds that they are only specialists in mental health. This annoys the disease psychiatrist. The late Dr Richard Hunter, one of the strongest adherents to the disease model, attacks this view in trenchant terms, 'Psychiatrists do not diagnose their patients like other doctors do. They discard four of their senses and literally play it by ear. It is the no-touch technique adapted to new purpose. Physical examination or laboratory investigation, which transformed medicine from guesswork and theory to fact and science, are spurned or positively discouraged. It is alleged that they deflect attention from study in depth of the patient's mind, and impede rapport' (Hunter, 1973). This is an interesting point – talking about symptoms in a formal way and examining the body systematically may not seem to be the best way to develop a good caring and sharing relationship with a patient – but it is regarded as essential in the disease model in order to avoid missing important pathology that could never be detected by the most perfect of professional relationships.

The same principles apply when carrying out an examination of the mental state (see Box 2.2). Although laboratory and other independent tests are not available to confirm the clinical findings the aim remains one of scientific objectivity. The examination of the mental state is the mental equivalent of the physical examination. The psychiatrist may have clues from the history as to which parts of the mental state are likely to be abnormal but must carry out the whole procedure as the history may be unreliable and there may be deliberate attempts to cover up the mental disturbance. The information he gets from the mental state examination is still not entirely objective (the adjectives 'soft' and 'hard' are often used to describe the differences in the quality of data) but it is still more reliable than the history.

SIMILARITIES IN MENTAL STATE AND PHYSICAL EXAMINATION

- Systematic examination of each organ system
- Systematic mental examination of behaviour, speech, thought and cognition
- Simple summary of abnormal findings (e.g. hypertension, hepatomegaly)
- Simple jargon to describe abnormal findings (e.g. grandiose delusions, flight of ideas)
- Provisional diagnosis once examination completed
- Diagnostic formulation once examination completed

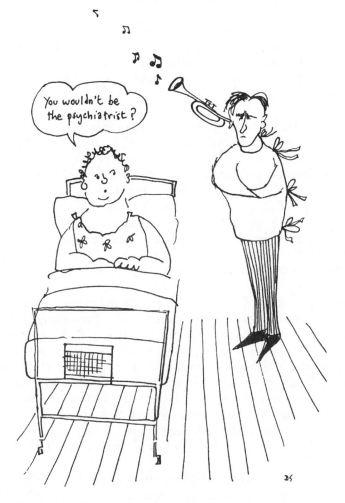

'They discard four of their senses and literally play it by ear'

Reporting the findings

In the same way that other doctors use a formal jargon to describe abnormal features on examination, such as 'generalized lymphadenopathy' for enlargement of lymph glands throughout the body, psychiatrists use a formal jargon to describe abnormal features in the mental state. This is called descriptive psychopathology or phenomenology, and its development owes a great deal to the work of Karl Jaspers (1963). The interviewer is trying to describe as objectively as possible the abnormal mental features elicited from his examination. By doing so he summarizes the findings in a form that is informative, concise and accurate, and certainly not an idiosyncratic assessment.

It is not sufficient merely to record the presence of an abnormality but to qualify it in the same way that a doctor will amplify a description such as hepatomegaly (enlarged liver) by saying how many fingerbreadths the liver is enlarged underneath the costal (rib) margin and whether it is hard or soft, smooth or knobbly.

For example, the judgement that events going on about you, and programmes on radio and television refer especially to you, is described in phenomenology as 'ideas of reference'. Similarly, the feelings of puzzlement and uncertainty that are common in the early stages of schizophrenia, when the patient suspects that something of great significance is happening but which he cannot yet identify, are called 'delusional mood'. The use of such terms greatly simplifies description in psychiatry and experience has shown that patients have a relatively small repertoire of abnormal mental functions in which certain phenomenological elements recur again and again. (A full list of these appears in the glossary of this book at the end).

The chief disadvantage of the information gathered in this way is that, like the history, it requires the patient's cooperation and depends largely on interpretation of what is said. Although an important part of the mental state examination is observation of the patient during the history and examination, it is rarely sufficient to assess a problem alone, so special procedures are necessary for mute and uncooperative patients. Nevertheless, by formalizing the subjective information from the patient the psychiatrist can summarize the disease in a few sentences. He is seldom able to make a diagnosis in a single word as can his medical colleagues, but his equivalent 'diagnostic formulation' is the most economical way he can communicate his findings.

Let us see how this works in practice. First of all let us look at the typical format of what students are taught as 'taking a case history' and in which we are using the disease model (Table 2.1). It is like building a house from the earliest stages.

Table 2.1:   Standard procedure for assessment using the disease model, linked to a useful analogy

1 Preparing the site	Taking the case history
2 Setting the foundation stones	Physical examination
3 Building the rooms	Examination of mental state
4 Decorating and plastering	Laboratory and other objective tests
5 Estate agent's specification	Diagnostic formulation

What information needs to be collected when 'taking the history'

Aquilina and Warner (2004) give an admirable summary of the basic skills necessary for this important assessment component of psychiatry. In order to carry out the history well the interviewer will '(i) be non-judgmental in attitude and approach, (ii), be interested in the patient and their concerns, (iii), listen to what the patient is saying and how they are saying it, (iv) observe the patient's appearance and behaviour, (v) be focused on the aims of the interview but also flexible, (vi) be in control of the interview yet able to allow spontaneity from the patient, encourage the discussion of difficult topics or feelings, (vii) stop the patient going into unnecessary detail or wandering off the point, (vii) be sensitive to their own and the patient's feelings by being aware of how the patient makes them feel and what effect they have on the patient' (Aquilina and Warner, 2004, p. 4).

Apart from the last point, which sometimes irritates the proponent of the disease model as it gets in the way of logical thought, all the others are consistent with the assessment of disease. Nonetheless, the interviewer has to engage the subject actively in this task to get the best returns of information and careful listening is an essential component of this. In the first part of the history – often described as 'main complaint' – the patient has the opportunity to explain, in his or her own words, exactly what constitutes the problem in their eyes and how it has developed. The views expressed may be completely wrong or exactly right, and the job of the assessor is to unravel this account by facilitating the patient so that a clear exposition of the problem is given in the patient's own words.

After that the barriers come down. The assessor is in control of the interview and has to do a lot in a short time. It is necessary to examine the family history in sequence (description of live and dead relatives, details of causes of death and any history of mental illness – so that family and genetic contributions to illness can be identified if present). This is followed by the personal history in which the birth circumstances and early life of the patient are recorded and details of schooling and performance obtained. Sexual history and marital relationships follow in sequence and details of wife (cohabitee) or other partners, and children, are also obtained. The previous personality – what the person was like before illness – is also asked about at this stage in the interview as it is important to find out to what extent the person has always been as at presentation or what changes have taken place in the recent past.

Because a great deal of information has to be obtained in this part of the interview the assessor has to be in firm control and may need to interrupt and change the flow of conversation to avoid unnecessary delay. This should not be interpreted as showing any lack of interest; it is just that there is so much that is irrelevant that could be said at this part of the examination and thereby waste valuable time.

The history of the present condition is then recorded in careful chronological detail, again with considerable control by the assessor and prompting at times to explore key points. The history is then followed by the physical and mental examination. The physical examination may or may not be carried out by the mental health professional (increasingly it is being left to other practitioners) but examination of the height, weight and appearance of the patient, and their presentation at interview can all be valuable even if a full examination is not carried out. The proponent of the disease model will need to be reassured that there is no physical disease present and will ensure that a recent full examination has already been carried out.

As explained earlier, the mental state examination is the equivalent of the physical one and goes through a standard procedure. The behaviour of the subject is described and their thoughts examined for signs of disorder. Of course, direct examination of thoughts cannot be carried out but much of thought is transferred into speech and analysis of speech content can tell a great deal about the person's thinking processes. The big advantage of recording exactly what the person has said helps others to interpret the significance of the statements.

Neuropsychological tests of cognition and memory complete the mental state examination. The ability to pay attention, to remember information and recall it after short intervals, an awareness of surroundings and recent events, are all parts of this assessment which help to decide on the diagnosis. Thus, for example, if the patient with the feelings of being possessed by aliens was being seen shortly after an operation in hospital and was somewhat confused at the time of assessment, this would throw a completely different light on the nature of the problem. The person who gives a long and rambling account of his condition at the beginning of the interview and then is shown to have gross memory disturbance at the end, could easily have a condition such as Korsakov's syndrome in which distortion of memory follows brain damage after long-term abuse of alcohol.

At the end of the interview the assessor will describe a diagnostic formulation in a few well-chosen sentences. As with the estate agent advertising a new house, the formulation advertises the patient's disorder in a highly specific way while still allowing the condition to be grouped with other disorders carrying the same label. An excellent diagnosis is one that explains everything in as few words as possible. Most psychiatric diagnoses are not as economical as this and a diagnostic formulation may be as much as a paragraph. For example, a person who presents with clinical symptoms of depression may need their problem to be put into context by a diagnostic formulation such as:

> 'A man of 25 with symptoms of depression following loss of esteem after failing an examination. He is currently feeling hopeless, lacking in self-esteem and has some biological features of depressive illness, including early morning waking and diurnal mood swing (feeling better as the day goes on). He is currently beginning to improve.'

Now that we have rehearsed the disease model let us see how it can work in actual practice. There are four stages in the process of establishing the nature of the disease and the first of these, the clinical assessment, is a critical one. Let us see if assessment using the model follows the advice given by Aquilina and Warner (2004). In the example (and others in this book) the interpretation is shown in brackets.

Assessment in practice

Young man of 24, referred to outpatient clinic from general practitioner. In the referral letter the essential elements are contained in two sentences. 'He has become much more withdrawn, and both his family and I think his personality has changed. He is much more suspicious of people and does not trust anybody; he does not trust me now because he has come repeatedly with complaints about his health and is not satisfied that I can find nothing physically wrong.'

Main complaint

The young man comes into the room for assessment. He looks nervous and the doctor gets up from his seat, comes towards him, shakes him by the hand and adopts a reassuring approach.

PSYCHIATRIST: 'I'm pleased to see you, Mr X; I'm Dr Y. I'm a psychiatrist. I know this may be a bit difficult for you coming here and I will be asking you quite a few questions. What I really need to do is to get an overall picture of how you are today and what might need to be done. So please excuse me if I ever have to interrupt you as I want to be able to advise you what needs to be done by the time we finish. But first I wonder if you could say how you see the main problem.'

PATIENT: (looking furtive) 'What problem? I don't know what you mean.'

PSYCHIATRIST: 'Well, the sort of thing that you might want help with. Something that may be troubling you?'

PATIENT: (after a pause) 'You can't help me. I need the police. Those people outside want to kill me. They're everywhere; they're taking over my mind as well. For all I know they've got at you too. How do I know?' (He falls silent).

INTERPRETATION: *This is a bonus for the assessment as important information has been disclosed right at the beginning. An important delusion is suspected, probably a paranoid delusion associated with the notion that he is being controlled (passivity). See Glossary for further information.*

PSYCHIATRIST: (realizing that this is a crisis point in the interview as it could end prematurely if he handles it wrongly) 'I can see this really is a problem. Don't bother to tell me anything else about this at the moment. I wonder if you could tell me some background information, not about you but about your family.'

PATIENT: (suspiciously) 'Why the family?'

PSYCHIATRIST: 'Well, as I said at the beginning I just want to get an overall picture. So I just want to get a feel of your background. Tell me about your father. What was he like?'

The conversation continues; the following information is written down by the psychiatrist. (He could do this later but he would like to get some comments *verbatim*).

Family history

Father 54, inventor. Has only had one major success, a patented can-opener, and has lived on the income from this for much of his life. Always isolated, few friends; preoccupied with pollution and healthy food. Has never trusted other people. On one occasion in the past felt his landlord was trying to harass him into leaving his rented property and his general practitioner asked for a psychiatric opinion. Would not accept treatment and compulsory admission to hospital was considered inappropriate. Since then has been suspicious of general practitioners and rarely consults them. *Interpretation: Father may have had a paranoid psychotic episode in the past and may also have a paranoid personality disorder. These features are part of what has been called the 'schizophrenia spectrum' which is often found in the families of those who have schizophrenia.* Mother, 50, divorced from husband five years ago. Quick-tempered, gregarious, never able to adjust to husband's self-imposed isolation and paranoia and left him for another man.

Patient an only child. Apart from father, a paternal uncle suffered from a mental illness thought to be schizophrenia. Had many admissions to hospital and committed suicide by jumping from a 10-storey building at the age of 49. *Interpretation: The information that another blood relative appears to have had schizophrenia or schizophreniform (schizophrenia-like) illnesses. May be relevant to patient's own condition as schizophrenia is transmitted partly by genetic factors.*

The psychiatrist has been successful in getting the patient on to more neutral territory, and continues with the details of the patient's early life.

PSYCHIATRIST: 'Can I move on to your own life. Where were you born?'

PATIENT: 'Why do you want to know that? What's that got to do with me now?'

PSYCHIATRIST: 'Sorry to trouble you about this. It may be quite unnecessary but I just need to get a picture of your background. I won't be mentioning it again unless it seems especially relevant.'

The man is reassured to some extent and the psychiatrist continues with the personal history.

Personal history

Born in an industrial town in the south of England. No birth problems, early development difficulties or childhood illnesses apart from measles. *Interpretation: No physical problems present in early life which might predispose him to psychiatric disorder.* Local primary and secondary schools, no special abilities, left at 16. Worked as a bookshop assistant for five years, eventually sacked because of poor time-keeping. Said he had lost interest in this work and 'could not be bothered as it did not mean anything to me'. Has not tried to get a job since but feels he has special abilities and the Government might ask him to work for them at some point in the future. Lives with father. Little contact with him, but he regards this as satisfactory and does not want to have a closer relationship. Has no close friends and little contact with women. 'I've never had a girlfriend, I've just had occasional sex with prostitutes.' Has no wish to get married or have any closer relationships with women.

Previous personality

Has always been a 'loner'. Regards other people as potentially threatening and finds it best to stay away from them. Used to collect stamps; no longer does so but regards his collection as special, and regards it as more important than any of his personal relationships. *Interpretation: The patient shows definite evidence of schizophrenia and schizoid personality disorder as described in the tenth revision of the International Classification of Disease (ICD-10) (World Health Organization, 1992). The combination of eccentricity, lack of emotional warmth and confiding relationships, and a preference for solitary activities are all typical features of this personality type.*

History of present condition

Over past two years increasingly concerned that people have been trying to harm him. When asked to explain this he said that the problems all began when the traffic lights at the crossroads outside his house ceased to work for a few days. Almost immediately afterwards he developed the notion that other people were following him and came to the conclusion that the traffic light failure was a deliberate signal to 'these people'. *Interpretation: delusional perception described.*

Claimed he could recognize these people because they communicated by technique which involved jangling loose change inside their pockets. He was therefore able to detect these people when they were standing in bus queues or in the street. In the past six months claimed these people were communicating with him in special ways. 'They can read my mind. They are aliens from another planet. They want to kill me so that they can take over my body in the same way they have taken over the bodies of all the other people who are following me. They won't be satisfied until they have taken me over completely. Have you got it? They're bloody f****** aliens, you've got to stop them. I know you don't believe me, no-one does, but its true.' *Interpretation: History indicates paranoid delusions and auditory hallucinations, and somatic delusions (body being controlled).*

The main part of this history has been completed. Already we have a great deal of information but we need to examine the young man more closely. There is also a worry that the patient is getting overwhelmed and excited by the questions and we need to get back on neutral ground.

PSYCHIATRIST: 'Thank you, that has been very helpful. Now I would just like to check your physical health by examining you.'

PATIENT: 'What do you want to do that for. Are you expecting to find the aliens?'

PSYCHIATRIST: 'I've got no idea. Its just that I need to check you are physically well. Just so I can get a full picture of the problem. We have to do this with everyone we see to make sure we can give you a clean bill of health'.

Physical examination

Tall, thin man, weight 69 kg, 1.8 m tall. No abnormalities noted in cardiovascular, respiratory, gastrointestinal or neurological systems.

Mental state examination

Behaviour: Extremely suspicious during interview, looking furtively about the room, became very agitated when he thought he heard someone walking past and jangling change outside in the corridor.

Speech: Talk intense and hesitant as though he was afraid of being overheard. Much of talk irrelevant, some speech difficult to follow (e.g. 'I know they can read my mind. Did you hear that noise? That tells me they are reading it now. I know I have the answer. The lights are off; they must go on again. They can kill me now if they want. I have my sword but I will not defend myself'). *Interpretation: Shows thought disorder typical of schizophrenia with lack of obvious connection between sentences (Knight's move).*

Thought content: Convinced that aliens controlled his mind and could pick up his thoughts and make him think what they wanted him to think. 'I can be part of them. They know my mind; they are in my mind. I must do exactly what they say. They are in control.' *Interpretation: Shows the phenomenon of 'passivity' together with gross thought disorder (including thought broadcasting and thought control with thought insertion). The belief that his mind is an empty vessel which is controlled by an alien force and that there is nothing he can do about it is one of the characteristic features of schizophrenia.* Perception: Hears the voices of aliens both telling him to do things, and also talking about him amongst themselves. They say things like 'he's not doing what we want; he must be half asleep. We'll have to wake him up.' Believes the voices come from space or possibly from another planet. Has never seen the aliens. *Interpretation: Has auditory hallucinations (i.e. the perception of hearing voices without the obvious stimulus of the voice). Some of these voices describe him in the third person and this is typical of schizophrenia.*

Cognition: Able to remember a name and address after five-minute recall and to do simple calculations such as subtracting seven from a hundred and subsequent subtractions of seven from the number produced. Is up to date with world affairs but not with local ones. Knows the date, time and place of interview. *Interpretation: He shows no significant intellectual impairment and is orientated in time and space.*

Diagnostic formulation: 'A young man with an apparent schizoid or schizotypal personality disorder who has become excessively suspicious, with auditory hallucinations and thought disorder, believing that his mind is being controlled by aliens. These symptoms are experienced in clear consciousness and the provisional diagnosis is that of paranoid schizophrenia (ICD-10 – Code 20.0; DSM-IV – 295.30).

We now look at whether the history has been obtained correctly using Aquilina and Warner's seven rules.

Rule 1. Non-judgmental in attitude and approach. I think we can approve the psychiatrist in this area. He (or she) (more often a she in today's mental health services) has been careful not to make any loaded comments that could be interpreted negatively by the patient. The patient is highly sensitive and can be upset by even neutral comments so great care has to be taken to keep him engaged. The disease model, which at its core regards everyone as being basically the same but having different illnesses affecting their mental function, is a non-judgmental model.

Rule 2. Being interested in the patient and their concerns. This can be a difficult problem in mental health. When someone like our patient has bizarre and strange beliefs it is frequent for them to want reinforcement from others. In order to maintain a reasonable level of cooperation psychiatrists often feel they have to collude with the patient to some extent. However, this is not always necessary. One of the mistakes that students sometimes make in assessing someone who seems to have an unequivocal severe mental illness is to assume that the patient is completely out of touch with reality and is not aware of 'normal' events and interactions. In fact, most people with schizophrenia are much more aware than we often give them credit for. As McCabe (2004) has noted '(schizophrenic) patients recognize that others do not agree with their delusional claims and are not persuaded by the justification they provide for these claims. Importantly, they recognize their own and others' discomfort at the disagreement this causes.' So it may not be necessary to collude, and our psychiatrist has given no indication of belief or rejection in the patient's alien explanations during the interview.

Rule 3. Listen to what the patient is saying and how they are saying it. This rule is followed closely by all aspirants to the disease model. Right from the opening phase of the interview it has been clear that there is something awry in the patient's thinking and this recognition (see the interpretation sections) has guided the interview.

Rule 4. Observe the patient's appearance and behaviour. This has again been followed. Right from the beginning of the interview the psychiatrist has noted that the patient is suspicious and uncomfortable and has tried to compensate for this by being both solicitous and friendly.

Rule 5. Be focused on the aims of the interview but also flexible. There is a clear focus on essential elements in the disease model and at some point in the assessment these have to be completed. The order is not absolutely essential but it is important to get the case history obtained as early as possible as this is such a valuable guide. In this example the physical examination was carried out a little earlier than usual. It broke up the interview but this was probably wise as the questioning was in danger of creating more suspicion and there was a danger of rejection and early termination of the assessment.

Rule 6. Be in control of the interview yet able to allow spontaneity from the patient, with encouragement of the discussion of difficult topics or feelings, while stopping the patient going into unnecessary detail or wandering off the point. This has been carried out as part of a delicate balancing act throughout the interview. The patient needs to be drawn out into expressing his thoughts, beliefs, interpretations and fears, but not in a way that loses control of the interview.

Rule 7. Be sensitive to your own and the patient's feelings by being aware of how the patient makes you feel and what effect you have on the patient. This is a difficult task in this instance, because the patient has an unusual way of interpreting his world and it takes time to understand it. However, we can give some indication of approval for the friendly, but detached, way in which the psychiatrist has kept this sensitive man engaged.

The rigidity of the disease model – the need to examine every person using the same basic approach – is often seized on by opponents of the disease model to illustrate that its practitioners do not care about people, they only subsume them into cases that they blindly assess in a common depersonalized and detached manner. This criticism is dismissed easily. A detective is at work here, trying to find a pathological needle hidden somewhere in a healthy haystack and, like all good detectives, has to look for clues that may not be immediately apparent to others. The need to examine every part of the patient's problem systematically, the detective's equivalent of 'leaving no stone unturned', ensures that nothing is left out.

Although the diagnosis may appear clear at this stage (it looks as though the patient has schizophrenia) it is only a provisional diagnosis (as are many diagnoses of physical disease after clinical examination). There are several other conditions that could give rise to a similar clinical picture, including the abuse of drugs such as amphetamines and LSD, or, more rarely, physical disease such as temporal lobe epilepsy. These conditions will have to be excluded before the diagnosis of paranoid schizophrenia is concluded as the definitive one.

The reader will note from this history and assessment that each element is interpreted, mainly in the shorthand of psychiatric description to aid communication, and that the assessment concentrates on those phenomena that are demonstrated (overt), not those which are hidden or unconscious (covert). The assessment is a rich information gathering exercise, carried out courteously but firmly. It prepares the way well for the next stage.

STAGE 2 – IDENTIFICATION OF PATHOLOGY

Clinical medicine cannot be practised well without other independent evidence that either confirms or refutes the diagnostic hints derived from clinical examination. The science of pathology is an essential handmaiden to good practice, and a range of investigations from simple estimations of haemoglobin concentration, electrolytes and liver function tests (from blood), to more complex tests such as computer assisted tomography (CAT) and magnetic resonance imaging (MRI) scans of different parts of the body, and examination of tissues obtained by biopsy or surgical removal, all help to hone the diagnosis, select treatment and predict prognosis.

But we have to be honest. In mental illness this part of assessment is more difficult than is physical medicine, because most mental disorder is not accompanied by obvious physical pathology. It is the demonstration of the specific features of schizophrenia described in the previous section, particularly the phenomenon of passivity, that helps to substitute for laboratory tests and clinches the diagnosis of schizophrenia. Of course this is not without risk; patients may simulate the diagnostic features of a disorder (called factitious disorder), or may only have them for such a short time that they do not qualify for a schizophrenic diagnosis, but this is no reason to decry them. It is remarkable that the symptoms of schizophrenia are virtually the same in all cultures and all races; people are not the same but illnesses are.

Still, laboratory tests can help. We are not quite at the stage when brain scans are standard investigations in schizophrenia but there is now clear evidence of abnormalities in the brains of some schizophrenic patients. These can be demonstrated by showing expansion of the ventricles (spaces between parts of the brain filled with fluid), which indicates reduction in the brain tissue surrounding these spaces. The lower parts of the brain, particularly a part called the hippocampus, may be the key abnormal structure (Harrison, 2004). There are also changes in function that can be identified using these special approaches collectively called *imaging*. Even the passage of an auditory hallucination through the brain can be identified using this approach (Shergill *et al.*, 2004) and so before long it may be possible to corroborate the patient's account of symptoms with independent evidence.

Genetic factors, as we have noted, are also important in many mental illnesses but their influence is not a straightforward one. Increasingly there is evidence that many of the conditions commonly labelled as severe mental illness, such as schizophrenia, bipolar disorder and severe autistic disorders, are neurodevelopmental ones and can also be linked to intellectual disability as there are cognitive impairments in all of them (Morgan *et al.*, 2012; Owen *et al.*, 2011; Owen, 2012). This also gives scope for another science linked to the disease model, neuropsychology, as often quite complex tests are needed to identify the abnormalities. Thus we have an interaction between the genotype, the genetic characteristics of a person, the characteristics of expression of the gene which are also heritable (epigenetics), and the phenotype, the combination of genotype, epigenetic factors and interaction with the environment. In psychiatry the notion of the endophenotype, a physiological, biochemical, endocrine, neuropsychological or other component of the disease (Gottesman and Gould, 2003), has also been a valuable one as any one endophenotype can be involved in genetic analysis. When opponents of the disease model say the variation in the expression of mental symptoms is so great it cannot be described in biological terms they are overlooking the tremendous breadth of these new approaches.

Mental symptoms may also be the precursors of physical disease and are therefore more sensitive detectors than more conventional tests. Von Economo's disease, for example, is a form of encephalitis that was first described in 1917 and became an epidemic in the 1920s before apparently dying out. Tiredness and extreme withdrawal (stupor) alternated with confusion and excitement in the acute phase and there was often nothing abnormal found on physical examination. The later development of the disorder occurred many years later after apparent return to normality following the acute illness. The disease associated with reduced functioning in the parts of the brain concerned with coordinating movement and posture (Parkinson's disease) emerged 20 years or more after the original episode. It would be easy to regard these two phases as separate illnesses but they are part of the same disease process. The mental symptoms may be an important clue to the presence of a disease and it is up to the doctor to describe them accurately and intimately rather than dismiss them as irrelevant.

STAGE 3 – THE NATURAL HISTORY (COURSE) OF THE SYNDROME

By taking the natural history of a disease (i.e. its course from beginning to end in the absence of treatment) into account, it is possible to improve the sensitivity of diagnosis. Thus it is now established that some people develop some (usually), or all (occasionally) of the symptoms of schizophrenia for very short periods only. Such illnesses are now called 'schizophreniform' (i.e. have the appearance of schizophrenia without necessarily being schizophrenia). Thus to acquire the diagnosis of paranoid schizophrenia in ICD-10 it is necessary for the symptoms to 'have been clearly present for most of the time during a period of one month or more' (World Health Organization, 1992). For those with shorter episodes other diagnoses are available such as *acute polymorphic psychotic disorder*.

Of course the natural history may be an intermittent or irregular one with no obvious pattern. But even here there can be important clues from the history. There is another rare but important disease, acute intermittent porphyria, which presents as severe attacks of abdominal pain and confusion and which has been alleged to be the cause of the mental illness shown by George III at the end of the eighteenth century (MacAlpine and Hunter, 1969), now made famous in the film *The Madness of King George*. The attacks of porphyria may be provoked by certain drugs such as barbiturates. Even quite common disorders such as recurrent anxiety may be associated with porphyria (Patience *et al.*, 1994).

STAGE 4 – DETERMINING THE CAUSE AND SELECTING RATIONAL TREATMENTS

By this stage in the assessment process our analogous disease model house is complete and almost ready for sale. The cause of the disease would be a tremendous bonus in understanding but for most mental illnesses is not available. For some organic conditions – Korsakov's psychosis (a form of dementia caused by alcohol poisoning), and for Alzheimer's disease – the cause is clear but for others it remains unclear. This is not a reason for dismissing the disease model; the jigsaw may be incomplete but the important picture can be seen. It is likely that genetics may be of assistance with many mental conditions. Genetic studies of all diseases are necessary to establish the relative importance of environmental and constitutional factors in the causation of illness. These interact so that even when there is an apparently clear environmental cause the disorder may still be influenced by hereditary factors. This has been shown with both schizophrenia and manic depressive (affective) psychoses, in which the standard technique of the geneticist, the study of the disease in monozygotic or identical (derived from a single cell) and dizygotic or nonidentical (derived from two separate cells) twins, reared together or apart, has revealed a high genetic loading. If the illness is hereditary, there is a greater risk of the second twin developing the illness if he or she is monozygotic. As the monozygotic twin has exactly the same genes as his co-twin (i.e. is technically a clone) the higher rate in these twins can only be explained by the disease having a hereditary basis.

Once all these stages of the disease model have been established, treatment often follows without any further knowledge being necessary, as in our young man with schizophrenia. But as we have found already, all too few of the mental illnesses we come across can be analysed in this comprehensive way. In the incomplete cases the doctor using the disease model adopts the empirical approach. He gives the most effective treatment known for the clinical syndrome he has identified if he knows that its natural history follows a chronic course, or he may do nothing if he knows that the condition has a good outcome. He will determine which treatments are most effective through the means of the randomized controlled trial and other similar enquiries that will lead to better 'evidence-based medicine'. There is no reason why mental disorders should have different rules for deciding on management. Clinical trials are often criticized by those who disapprove of the disease model in psychiatry because they are alleged 'to make people into guinea pigs', testing them without proper informed consent being obtained and without their doctors really believing that it is an appropriate treatment for the individual. Doctors involve patients in such studies because they 'feel torn by their obligations to individual patients and to society at large, and they may even have got the impression, perhaps hyped up by advocates of evidence based medicine, that they are obliged to participate in research for the common good' (Edwards *et al.*, 1998).

However, this is a criticism of the process, not the principle. Most of the advances in medicine made in the past fifty years have involved the randomized controlled trial, beginning with the demonstration that smoking causes lung cancer (Doll and Bradford Hill, 1950) and even if you regard these trials as evil, they are necessary evils and cannot be substituted. In any case, all the treatments described in the other models in this book have also been tested, more or less willingly, using this approach.

In this way conclusions can be made about the effectiveness of the treatment much more rapidly than knowledge gained by trial and error. The demonstration of an effective treatment may also help to discover some of the other stages in the disease model. For example, it is known that most patients with the clinical syndrome of schizophrenia are dramatically improved by treatment with one or more of the antipsychotic group of drugs (there are atypical and typical members) and will relapse if these drugs are withdrawn or reduced to half their original dose (Johnson *et al.*, 1987). The symptoms of schizophrenia are suppressed and yet other aspects of brain function are unchanged. This, according to the disease model, is evidence of a specific brain abnormality in schizophrenia, which is corrected by drug treatment. The abnormality is not entirely clear but all these drugs act by blocking the effects of a naturally occurring amine, dopamine, on certain brain sites (receptors) in the brain (Carlsson and Lindqvist, 1963).

There is abundant evidence in medicine of treatments that were shown to be effective long before it was known how they worked; and with these precedents the disease psychiatrist should have no qualms in defending the empirical approach. So the fuss that some people make over the use of electroconvulsive therapy (ECT) will not trouble him, for he is satisfied by the evidence of clinical trials that for some psychiatric conditions, particularly depressive psychosis (the diagnosis is important), ECT is a highly effective form of treatment and may be life-saving in someone with strong suicidal feelings associated with depression. The fact that a somewhat unusual form of treatment such as ECT is still given without knowing why it works is important for the scientist to elucidate but should not inhibit the therapist from giving it when its effectiveness has been demonstrated (Gregory *et al.*, 1985).

The critic may respond by claiming that the disease model is unjustified in assuming that all the psychiatric conditions over which it claims authority are diseases in the accepted sense. It is not good enough to presume that in time a bodily pathology will be found in such conditions as depression and schizophrenia. The demonstration of pathology should precede therapeutic intervention, particularly for those procedures such as prefrontal leucotomy.

This criticism can be countered on empirical grounds – if we waited until we were certain what was wrong before starting treatment most current therapy would have to cease forthwith but it also brings up the question of the dividing line between disease and non-disease in psychiatry. This is not so easy to answer, but most accept Scadding's view (1967) that to qualify for a disease label a medical condition must be biologically disadvantageous. In other words, it must either harm the individual or reduce his or her capacity to reproduce.

Setting boundaries for the disease model

Taking this as the criterion for disease several psychiatric conditions can be excluded and the boundary between normality and illness becomes defined. The condition 'hysteria' which is impossible to diagnose except by exclusion of other pathology, is not included as formal mental illness. The classical symptoms of 'conversion and 'dissociation' are said by psychodynamic psychiatrists to be unconsciously motivated and secure some advantage for the victim, commonly called 'secondary gain'. Quite apart from the inability to assess unconscious motivation in a formal examination of the mental state, which necessarily implies that no conscious indication of it will be shown to the examiner, the idea that a symptom produces some advantage is incompatible with the disease concept. Hysteria as a diagnosis, therefore, is not permissible, and no longer appears in the diagnostic nomenclature. There are many psychiatric disorders which grade, apparently imperceptibly, between normality and illness, but the disease model can categorize them adequately. Mental handicap, for example, includes people who are so severely retarded that they are incapable of performing independently the simplest tasks necessary to ensure survival, and also those who can live independently but can only take up simple occupations because of their limited intelligence. The latter would not come into the disease category of mental subnormality; whereas the first group would, according to Scadding's criteria. Probably 'mental handicap' should best be used as a term to describe intellectual functioning, and the term 'disease' involved when there is identifiable brain pathology, as is the case for most people with very severe mental handicap.

There are several other approaches to practice that accompany the disease model. The emphasis on adequate diagnosis and formal classification of psychiatric conditions means that patients are placed in groups and common methods of treatment sought for them. The critic immediately responds by condemning the crudity of a system that regards patients as cases and not as unique individuals who should be dealt with on an individual basis. The disease model's proponents dismiss this as emotive nonsense, arguing that if every patient's condition is regarded as unique in all respects then psychiatry is not a medical discipline but a lottery in which we learn something from each patient but forget it all when we move to the next one. The combination of characteristics that make up a mental disorder is unique, but there are common features that, in a good classification, are found in all other patients within the group, and by using the body of information derived from previous knowledge of the disorder, together with basic scientific information from neuropsychology, genetics, brain scans (currently still very limited in the individual case), and biology, a more logical and effective system of management can be chosen. As Rutter and Gould (1985) have pointed out in explaining the usefulness of classification in a wider context, it is disorders we are attempting to classify, not people.

Another important facet of the disease model is that the patient is regarded as a passive recipient of treatment. Although the onset and course of the illness is frequently influenced by what the person does, by the time the disease is manifest he is a helpless victim needing external intervention. Just as pneumonia needs antibiotics to reinforce the body's defences against the bacteria that are multiplying rapidly in the lung, the psychiatric patient needs a similar specialist treatment temporarily to replace his normal coping mechanisms. These mechanisms have presumably been employed at an earlier stage in the illness and have demonstrably failed, otherwise the patient would not be seeking specialist advice. Moral exhortations and encouragement are therefore irrelevant to the treatment given according to the disease model. The brain is not functioning properly and the focus of treatment should be directed to the seat of disorder. It is good manners to be considerate to the patient and to respect his rights, and good cooperation means that the patient is more likely to adhere to the treatment prescribed, but it is not an essential part of therapy. The best treatment is the 'magic bullet' – to use the phrase of Paul Ehrlich, one of the first to treat disease scientifically – that eradicates the focus of disease without harming any healthy parts of the body.

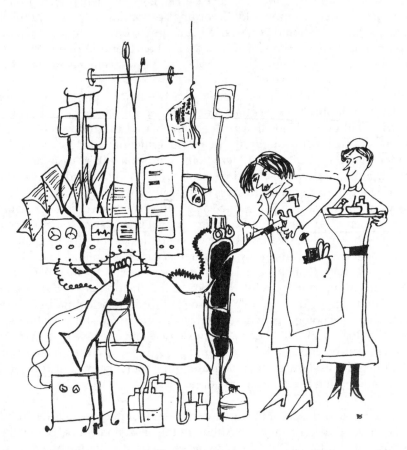

' . . . the patient is regarded as a passive recipient of treatment'

As the patient's own part in treatment is relatively small it is not possible to blame the patient for failure to respond on the grounds that he or she is showing resistance or some other psychodynamic mechanism (a view that is looked on sceptically by those using the disease model as it is incapable of verification). So if a patient with an agreed diagnosis fails to respond to a particular treatment that is normally effective for that illness, then more powerful treatments are selected or the diagnosis is questioned, instead of making the patient responsible for the lack of response. To quote Dr Hunter again 'patients are characterized by epithets which insult their personality and intelligence. Their sufferings are denied by being described in terms of "will not" where body doctors would say "can not" and try to discover why. No other specialty blames illness – and therapeutic failures on patients'.

Attitudes of doctors in the disease model

It follows naturally that if the patient has a dependent role in the disease model the doctor has an authoritative one. As the psychiatrist is approached as an expert for advice he accepts this role and acts accordingly. He responds to criticism that he is being patronizing or condescending by saying that the authoritarian role has accompanied good medicine throughout the centuries. If the patient has faith in the doctor and accepts his judgement, treatment will be more effective. It is also argued that most patients prefer their doctor to be an authoritarian, rather than presenting a phoney equality that only makes patients feel uncomfortable. If the phrase 'Trust me, I'm a doctor', has lost some of its message in recent years it is perhaps because too many doctors have been distracted from the disease model in their work.

The authority of the doctor also affects his relationships with other members of the psychiatric team. A definite hierarchy exists, with the doctors taking precedence over other professional workers such as nurses, psychologists, social workers and occupational therapists. This is because the doctors alone have sufficient training in both medicine and psychiatry to both examine the mental and physical state, and to exercise appropriate clinical responsibility, as Craddock and his colleagues argue (2008). The psychiatrist in the disease model does not take kindly to working in a multidisciplinary psychiatric team in which all members are alleged experts and insist on the democratic process.

As psychiatric illness often mimics or foreshadows physical illness it is right and proper for the doctor to be the chief decision maker and head of the team. Following assessment he may delegate responsibility to a greater or lesser degree but will always maintain clinical responsibility for the patient, as only he or she has the breadth of knowledge and skills to carry out this role.

Compulsory treatment

The disease model can also defend the need for occasional compulsory admission and treatment. Psychiatric illness is due to disordered brain function, and as the brain is concerned with higher elements of consciousness

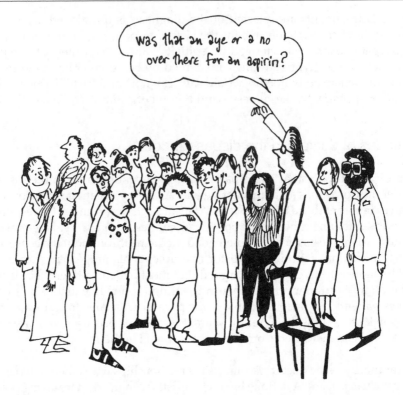

' . . . all members are alleged experts and insist on the democratic process'

such as judgement and insight it is to be expected that often these elements become impaired. If they do, and if the disease can be arrested or cured by treatment, it is appropriate for the doctor to act on behalf of the patient even if it is against the patient's wishes. Just as the first-aid worker does not need consent to practise artificial respiration on the unconscious patient dragged from a swimming pool, the psychiatrist does not necessarily require consent to treat a life-threatening mental illness that has altered the patient's judgement so that he acts and thinks abnormally.

The concept of abnormality is derived from the patient's previous level of functioning before illness and from knowledge of the psychiatric disorder. For example, the so-called manic phase of bipolar disorder is very frequently accompanied by lack of insight. During this phase the patient is overactive and frequently believes himself to be superior to others around him. He can develop grandiose ideas or delusions that he is a brilliant doctor himself, owns a large organization such as a bank or has supernatural powers. If he is likely to act on these delusions by spending thousands of pounds he does not have or attempting to fly like Superman from high buildings, admission to hospital is essential and continued community treatment is far too risky. Orders for compulsory admission allow a person's liberty to be taken away if he or she suffers from an illness that is liable to affect health adversely or be a danger to others. It is therefore appropriate to treat such patients against their wishes, knowing from previous experience of this disorder that they will return to normal after treatment.

Abnormality of this sort, according to the disease model, is quite different from social abnormality. Compulsory admission is not carried out just because a patient is acting in an antisocial manner. It is true that some illnesses may demonstrate antisocial behaviour as one feature of the disorder but the decision to treat compulsorily is made on the evidence of illness, not on behaviour alone. This is why psychiatrists will not accept patients as ill just because they are aggressive. If they are acting antisocially and are not ill they should be dealt with by the process of law. The disease model does not therefore accept the notion that a condition such as dangerous and severe personality disorder, recently introduced by the UK government (Home Office and Department of Health, 1999), can be regarded as a disease without further evidence, and indeed, such evidence is still awaited (Tyrer *et al.*, 2010).

The disease model in psychiatry is presented as a logical and well-tried approach to illnesses of the mind. It is a scientific model and relies on testable theories rather than woolly speculation. As with all science, theories are tested and retested until the best working hypothesis is found, only for this to be rejected when it is shown to be inadequate in the light of new knowledge (Popper, 1963). The model takes away the mythology and mystique from mental illness and replaces them with a rational approach that allows psychiatry to come together with other medical disciplines and share in the advances that they have made.

Medical students who read the above account will understand this approach much better than others who are not trained in the same way as doctors. The examination of the patient's mind is similar in many ways to the examination of the body. The main difference is, of course, that we cannot examine the mind physically in the same way we can someone who has a broken leg or a pain in the stomach. You therefore examine the mind indirectly, by analysing some of the most important products of the mind, primarily thoughts expressed in the form of speech. In addition to this the examiner also observes the patient and notes any unusual behaviour in exactly the same way as the doctor examining a patient for a medical illness would observe abnormal physical features such as a mottled complexion, an unusual walk or a skin rash, whether or not it is complained of by the patient. The combination of clinical inquiry eliciting the main psychopathological features together with the keen observation of the detective enables the doctor to come to a diagnosis. This diagnosis is an exact description of a condition shared by many other patients and has the great advantage of allowing efficient communication between professionals. A good diagnosis gives an indication of cause, the main clinical features, the recommended treatment and the likely prognosis.

DEFENCE OF THE DISEASE MODEL

The practitioner of the disease model is often criticized for failing to see the whole person in his task of identifying a so-called disease in the patient's mind. This criticism is easily dismissed: the good medical doctor does not lose sight of the person when diagnosing hypertension in a 45-year-old bank manager. He has to take notice of this in his recommendations to the person after the high blood pressure has been identified. Advice about work and lifestyle are part of the management of hypertension but the main diagnostic process has to take place independently of this. The doctor has to be satisfied that the high blood pressure is a persistent feature and just not a temporary phenomenon, that it has no immediately treatable cause (i.e. it is essential hypertension), and whether there are particular reasons for not prescribing certain treatments compared with others.

These kinds of decisions are clinical ones and exactly the same decisions have to be made by the psychiatrist operating the disease model. Unfortunately the adjective 'clinical' in this setting is often regarded as a rude word. It implies that the psychiatrist has lost his or her humanity, and merely looks at patients as disease objects. When making an assessment of a patient with suspected schizophrenia there are no special advantages in being especially sensitive to the person's individuality. Of course each person with schizophrenia is unique, and so is every case of essential hypertension, but the personal characteristics of the patient should not interfere with the investigation of the disease. The psychiatrist who sends our patient with suspected schizophrenia for an electroencephalogram (EEG) or a neuromagnetic imaging (NMI) scan is not being inhumane or uncaring; he is merely trying to find important treatable causes of the patient's symptoms that might well be forgotten if the main assessment was only of the patient's innermost feelings and how he was reacting to his disorder.

The critic may also reply that whereas diagnoses such as schizophrenia are sometimes appropriate for the disease model, others are quite unsuitable. This criticism is also rebutted. Careful studies show that almost all mental illness, ranging from anxiety following an unpleasant stress to major psychoses such as schizophrenia and manic depression (affective psychoses), are associated with biochemical, neuropharmacological and hormonal changes. These changes can be measured and are often indicative of pathology. In the broader sense they can therefore be regarded as diseases and the fact that we cannot identify a part of the brain that is pathological at the present state of our knowledge, does not mean that no such change exists. Indeed, schizophrenia was identified at the turn of the century and not found to be associated with any physical disease. It is only in the past 15 years that organic abnormalities have been found with mental patients suffering from this disorder.

So we can return to Eliot Slater's assertion that the physical approach is 'in line with the main front of biological advance' and is where psychiatry belongs. If we had failed to use the disease model we never would have discovered that general paralysis of the insane was caused by the syphilis spirochaete, that dementia of the Alzheimer's type is associated with certain characteristic neurofibrillary tangles in the brain that explain the death of brain cells, and that Huntington's chorea is a genetically determined disease. There are many more conditions that will soon join this group, and it is not unreasonable to think that all mental disorders will in time be shown to be diseases in the medically accepted sense, and at that eventually psychiatry and medicine will be as one.

REFERENCES

Aquilina, C. and Warner, P. (2004) *A Guide to Psychiatric Examination*. PasTest, Knutsford, Cheshire.

Craddock, N., Antebi, D., Attenburrow, et al. (2008) Wake-up call for British psychiatry. *British Journal of Psychiatry*, **193**, 6–9.

Carlsson, A. and Lindqvist, M. (1963) Effect of chlorpromazine or haloperidol on formation of 3-methoxytyramine and normetanephrine in mouse brain. *Acta Pharmacologica et Toxicologica*, **20**, 140–144.

Doll, R. and Bradford Hill, A. (1950) Smoking and carcinoma of the lung: a preliminary report. *British Medical Journal*, **2**, 739–748.

Edwards, S.J.L., Lilford, R.J. and Hewison, J (1998) The ethics of randomised controlled trials from the perspectives of patients, the public, and healthcare professionals. *British Medical Journal*, **317**, 1209–1212.

Gottesman, I.I. and Gould, T.D. (2003) The endophenotype concept in psychiatry: etymology and strategic intentions. *American Journal of Psychiatry*, **160**, 636–645.

Gregory, S., Shawcross, C.R. and Gill, D. (1985) The Nottingham ECT study: a double-blind comparison of bilateral, unilateral and simulated ECT in depressive illness. *British Journal of Psychiatry*, **146**, 520–524.

Harrison, P.J. (2004) The hippocampus in schizophrenia: a review of the neuropathological evidence and its pathophysiological implications. *Psychopharmacology*, **174**, 151–162.

Home Office and Department of Health (1999) *Managing Dangerous People with Severe Personality Disorder: Proposals for Policy Development*. Department of Health, London.

Hunter, R. (1973) Psychiatry and neurology: psychosyndrome or brain disease? *Journal of the Royal Society of Medicine*, **66**, 359–364.

Jaspers, K. (1963) *General Psychopathology*, translated by Hoenig, J. and Hamilton, M.W. Manchester University Press, Manchester.

Johnson, D.A., Ludlow, J.M., Street, K. and Taylor, R.D. (1987) Double-blind comparison of half-dose and standard-dose flupenthixol decanoate in the maintenance treatment of stabilised out-patients with schizophrenia, *British Journal of Psychiatry*, **151**, 634–638.

MacAlpine, I. and Hunter, R. (1969) *George III and the Mad Business*. Allen Lane, London.

McCabe, R. (2004) On the inadequacies of Theory of Mind explanations of schizophrenia: alternative accounts of alternative problems. *Theory and Psychology*, **14**, 738–752.

Morgan, V.A., Croft, M.L., Valuri, G.M., *et al.* (2012) Intellectual disability and other neuropsychiatric outcomes in high-risk children of mothers with schizophrenia, bipolar disorder and unipolar major depression. *British Journal of Psychiatry*, **200**, 282–289.

Owen, M.J. (2012) Intellectual disability and major psychiatric disorders: a continuum of neurodevelopmental causality. *British Journal of Psychiatry*, **200**, 268–269.

Owen, M.J., O'Donovan, M.C., Thapar, A. and Craddock, N. (2011) Neurodevelopmental hypothesis of schizophrenia. *British Journal of Psychiatry*, **198**, 173–175.

Royal College of Psychiatrists and National Institute for Mental Health in England (2005) *New Ways of Working for Psychiatrists: Enhancing Effective, Person-centred Services through New Ways of Working in Multidisciplinary and Multi-agency Contexts. Final Report 'But Not the End of the Story'*. Department of Health, London.

Patience, D.D., Blackwood, D.H.R., McColl K.E.L. and Moore, M.R. (1994) Acute intermittent porphyria and mental illness – a family study. *Acta Psychiatrica Scandinavica*, **89**, 262–267.

Popper, K. (1963) *Conjecture and Refutations: the Growth of Scientific Knowledge*. Routledge & Kegan Paul, London.

Rutter, M. and Gould, M. (1985) Classification. In: M. Rutter and L. Hersov (eds), *Child and Adolescent Psychiatry – Modern Approaches*. Blackwell Scientific Publications, Oxford.

Sargant, W. and Slater, E. (1954) *An Introduction to Physical Methods and Treatment in Psychiatry*. Livingstone, Edinburgh.

Scadding, J.E. (1967) Diagnosis: the clinician and the computer. *Lancet*, **ii**, 877–882.

Shergill, S.S., Brammer, M.J., Amaro, E., Williams, S.C.R., Murray, R.M. and McGuire, P.K. (2004) Temporal course of auditory hallucinations. *British Journal of Psychiatry*, **185**, 516–517.

Tyrer, P., Duggan, C., Cooper, S. *et al.* (2010) The successes and failures of the DSPD experiment: the assessment and management of severe personality disorder. *Medicine, Science and the Law*, **50**, 95–99.

World Health Organization (1992) *International Classification of Diseases*, 10th Edn. WHO, Geneva.

3

THE PSYCHODYNAMIC MODEL

'There are nine and sixty ways of conducting tribal lays, And every single one of them is right.'

Rudyard Kipling *In the Neolithic Age*

There are many misconceptions about the psychodynamic model, even supposing that a single model can be said to exist; and some suggest it may be more accurate to think of the psychodynamic approach as a particular style of clinical thinking. It follows from this that even among its adherents there is a good deal of argument over the essential elements of the psychodynamic approach, which comprises many quite different conceptions of theory and practice.

The variety of practice that comes broadly into the psychodynamic sphere of influence illustrates that, contrary to what some of its critics say, psychodynamic thinking has not stood still, fossilized, since the late nineteenth and early twentieth century, when its basic tenets were being developed by Freud, Jung, Adler and their followers. It has made many significant advances since, in terms of refining concepts, in making connections with other disciplines (notably biology and social science), and in new types of clinical practice.

It is true that there remain purists who have tended to disown some of the new developments; one of us, attending a conference which sought to show the useful interconnections between biological, social and psychodynamic models, heard a distinguished French psychoanalyst sum up the meeting by thundering that he had learned nothing new or of interest, and that the family therapists (he singled them out) must have had something wrong with their analytic training. Nevertheless we would identify family

Models for Mental Disorder: Conceptual Models in Psychiatry, Fifth Edition. Peter Tyrer.
© 2013 John Wiley & Sons, Ltd. Published 2013 by John Wiley & Sons, Ltd.

therapy, group therapy, many aspects of psychotherapy and counselling, much of the creative therapies (e.g. art therapy) and some interesting developments in organizational psychology (i.e. the psychological study of institutions) and consultative work as branches of the psychodynamic tree.

Amid all this, what is psychoanalysis? And who are the psychoanalysts? Psychoanalysis, which is synonymous with the theories of Sigmund Freud (1856–1939), Moravian physician and neurologist, relates to psychodynamic theory in roughly the way Darwinism relates to biology. It is not the whole story, and is not without controversy, but it is one of several fundamental tenets. People often classify psychotherapists, those who use the talking treatments, into behaviour therapists (including cognitive-behavioural therapists) and psychodynamic therapists, and the latter group are considered to be adherents of the general psychodynamic model, while noting that it uses several different concepts and approaches.

Psychodynamic therapists make use of psychoanalytic principles, but only a proportion of them will necessarily be trained analysts. Of the psychoanalytically trained psychotherapists, again only a proportion practise classical psychoanalysis, that is, with the patient talking from a recumbent position on a couch, with the psychoanalyst spending most of the time listening. Much psychoanalytic psychotherapy is conducted for training purposes (i.e. training other psychodynamic psychotherapists) but tends to be known nonetheless as 'being in therapy' by these trainees, which is a confusing notion. We consider training one thing, therapy another. Dynamic psychotherapy can be on a weekly basis for a few weeks or months; psychoanalysis may be daily for several years. Between these extremes are many variations.

Another feature of psychodynamic therapy for the purposes of this general introduction is the concept of supervision. The average house physician or house surgeon arrives on the first day of the first job with his bleep going as he struggles into a starched white coat, and supposedly knows everything. In a week or so, at a ward round, he is politely interrogated by the consultant about the surviving patients. The professional undertaking kosher psychodynamic psychotherapy, however, is expected to take his or her work, for years to come, to a psychodynamic psychotherapist for supervision, at which, session by session, every utterance of patient and therapist, every non-verbal action (e.g. being late, a yawn, a period of silence) is explored in depth for the light it may throw on the patient, the problem, the progress of the work and the therapist.

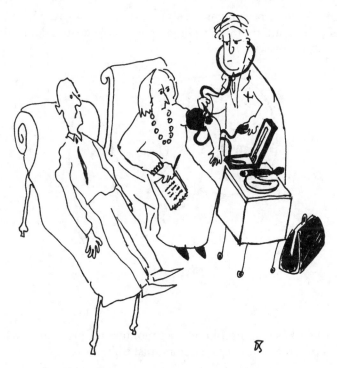

'psychoanalysis may be daily for several years'

IS IT TRUE? DOES IT WORK?

There is a great deal of truth in psychodynamic notions, but it is not the whole truth. It is also true that again and again it defies attempts to 'prove' it is effective, because 'it' varies so much, and it is difficult to define objective criteria for progress. On the one hand clinicians who pay attention to what their patients say and do and to their own personal reactions will find an intriguing face validity in the psychodynamic way of looking at things. On another hand, spending time attending to the meanings and feelings behind the superficial words of people in difficulties is also, in the words of a pragmatic and distinguished practitioner, 'a very civilized, humane service offered to another human being' (Wilson, 1986). Yet, on the third hand, psychodynamic psychotherapy is time-consuming and therefore expensive, and too easy, in a liberal, well-meaning sort of way, to suggest for everybody, even those who would be better off with, say, medicatioxn or behaviour therapy.

Nonetheless it is ridiculous simply to dismiss it as rubbish. (Interestingly, to do so illustrates the angry use of a metaphor for encapsulating the notion of dirt, dust, junk and other unwanted stuff best thrown away, which is *precisely* the sort of combination of real feelings plus usable abstractions with which psychodynamicists work.)

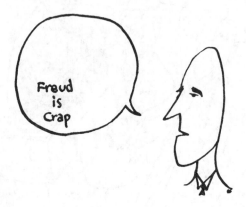

BASICS

Here are a few basic assumptions, or fundamental principles, which illustrate how a psychodynamic psychotherapist thinks.

BASIC PRINCIPLES OF PSYCHODYNAMICS
• The focus is the pattern of feelings • We are unaware of many influential feelings • A technically structured approach is needed to tap unconscious feelings • Important feelings manifest as emotional reactions to the therapist (transference) • As important are the therapist's reactions to the patient (countertransference) • The apparent moral neutrality of the therapeutic contract represents the therapist's efforts to be objective, not judgmental • Troubling feelings, inconsistencies, irrationalities are part of the universal balancing act involved in being human; it is imbalance that underlies emotional disorder • There is a constant interplay of complicated feelings (hence dynamic) with a 'final common outcome' at any time, as in a parallelogram of forces or in the neurophysiological concept of the final common path • Unconscious processes are influential in relationships of all sorts (e.g. artist and audience as well as doctor and patient) without either necessarily knowing why • Unconscious feelings find an important part of their expression in symbols: words, for example

Principle 1

The therapist's interest and clinical business is how the patient's feelings have led to problematic thinking and behaving.

Principle 2

Neither therapist nor patient can tell you immediately what these patterns of feelings are, because they are a complex mixture of things valued, things disliked, things only partially grasped, and things so elusive that they cannot be put into words at all. And when they are put into words, the words seem inadequate, not only intellectually but in terms of the feelings behind them. Moreover, both thoughts and feelings may be contradictory: the patient may like and dislike, or love and fear, certain people, things or situations, and indeed would need the skills of an accomplished poet or novelist to convey them with any felicity (see Principle 10). What the patient is aware of, or an attitude he or she adopts, is the tip of the iceberg of feelings, much of which is only partially conscious, or unconscious, but which is influential nonetheless.

The notion of the unconscious is fundamental to the concept of unperceived feelings, and to the psychodynamic model. The unconscious is hard to discuss without reaching for misleading analogies. In Freud's time, when nineteenth-century physics and engineering were at their peaks, the models for that which was beyond verbal description tended to be geological or hydraulic: pressures from within, held down by powerful forces, diverted by valves, leaking out like molten lava or a burst pipe, were the metaphors of the day.

In an earlier time, demons, angels and similar beings up there or down below were invoked for explaining the inexplicable. More recently, models for the mind have tended towards electronic circuits. At present we are moving into the quantum physics and chaos theory mode, and we may well wonder about the conceptual models of the future. An example of a model that misleads is the hydrodynamic, 'pressure cooker' model of stress, which may make people interpret uncomfortable feelings as internal forces that must be 'let out' one way or another. In fact, the relationship between such concepts and effective treatments is unclear.

A simpler concept for the 'unconscious', and one consistent with much psychodynamic thinking and therapy, connects conscious and observable verbal and non-verbal signals (words plus the minutiae of social behaviour) with internal feelings and images. Presented with any simple or complex stimulus (e.g. a phrase, an image or the first perception of another person) we can pursue a train of thought which can lead in unexpected directions. It may make unexpected connections, 'lighting up' pleasant or unwelcome images and associated feelings, some relevant, some irrelevant, or make the day-dreamer become alert with a start as something urgent and forgotten is recalled; perhaps the promise to make a phone call. It is likely that the sort of verbal connections that happen when one *free associates* in this way (the term and technique are those of the Swiss psychiatrist and psychoanalyst C.G. Jung) have some neurophysiological and neurochemical representation in the brain tracts and synaptic connections. It is also likely that such connections range from the entirely random, through those more or less habitual, to some predisposed by anatomy and evolution, and some triggered by matters currently important in our mental lives. The same may be true of dreams and fantasy. It is also probable that countless such connections are being made, interconnected and broken all the time as part of the brain's life and alertness, precipitated by stimuli from within and without which range from the most trivial (the feel of your bottom on the chair, now) to something more imperative (e.g. a knock at the door, or an idea for a novel). The buzzing brain, or what Charles Sherrington, the distinguished neurophysiologist, called 'an enchanted loom with millions of flashing shuttles', has many tasks to perform and, in modulating the sympathetic, parasympathetic and endocrine systems with cortical activity, is likely to file away much that is

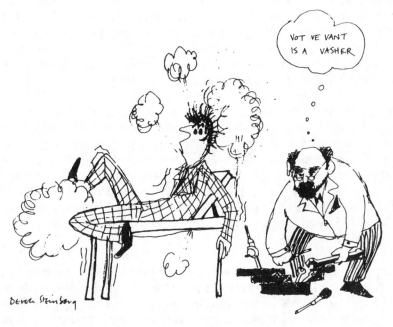

'...leaking out like molten lava or a burst pipe...'

inaccessible except in certain circumstances (e.g. relaxation, dreaming, psychoanalysis) and some that is easily available if we 'turn our minds' to it. This may be a more valid model than the idea of inner pressures or a murky dark sea in which strange denizens ('complexes') are imagined to swim or lurk.

Whatever model is preferred, however, the unifying idea is of substantial mental activity continuing outside our awareness, yet at the same time being able to influence our awareness. Opponents of the concept of the unconscious mind have suggested that the very notion is illogical – that something unconscious cannot be part of the mind. They may have a point, in that unconscious thought is perhaps an oxymoronic concept (on the basis that the accessible component of thinking is, by definition, a conscious process), but there is nothing inherently unsound in the notion of our thoughts and feelings being influenced by, or even driven by, internal psychophysiological processes.

Principle 3

It takes time and mental exploration to begin to convey these things. It also takes a trusting relationship in which the patient can feel comfortable enough to become aware of and admit to himself, let alone anyone else, such a range of thoughts, doubts and mixed feelings. These may include feelings of sexual attraction or burning resentment (or both) towards his or her relations, friends and others, doubts about personal abilities, ambitions of cosmic proportions, or other such unworthy or manic ideas. All this takes time, and because it can be tricky and uncomfortable, and in a sense undisciplined (i.e. chaotic, unsystematic, uncensored), it works best within a definitely agreed framework. Thus whatever does or does not go on within a session, it is for a fixed period at a definite and regular time and place. The rules of time and place provide the safe structure within which decidedly unsafe matters can be explored. Thus, any other sort of clinician may give popular patients frequent, long appointments and unpopular patients infrequent, short ones. The psychotherapist has technical reasons for keeping it the same come what may. (For example, an apparently reasonably self-confident person might fear his/her therapist did not like him/her if, after the therapist was mildly critical of them, they were a little late for the next appointment. But such things happen, and are allowed for in the psychotherapist's technology.)

Principle 4

The latter points to a most important and fundamental assumption: that in general the ideas and feelings that mess people up are a little like free radicals in chemistry, that is they tend to attach themselves to other people, or more precisely colour the image of the other person and therefore affect the relationship. Thus suppose your patient has reasons in his psyche to tend to be paranoid. This paranoia (used here as a portmanteau term for any number of complex and subtle feelings) may have emerged in a relationship with a parent, become part of his repertoire in growing up, influenced his relationship with his wife, got in the way in relationships at work, and now (after the honeymoon period of therapy is over, during which you were the nice, kind therapist) attaches itself to you. This is the essence of transference, and goes well beyond the popular conception of 'falling in love with the analyst'. The wish to murder the therapist is more likely, and more useful. It is this immediate resurrection of old relationships with which the therapist works. Which are the 'real' feelings? Characteristically there can be real but opposing feelings, formulated as ambivalence.

Principle 5

How are you to know that such feelings are there? The patient may well not tell you, particularly in the early stages, may reveal them later, or sometimes never. The experienced therapist is alert to his or her own feelings towards the patient. The whole point of the dynamic psychotherapist having a training which gives psychodynamic insight is that such feelings of his own will be examined as objectively as possible; the philosopher and psychiatrist Henri Ey gave this important notion (the objective observation of subjective feelings) philosophical and clinical respectability (Evans, 1972). It is important to appreciate that intellectual insight is not enough; the powerful, mixed and varying feelings that the patient in due course beams towards anyone who listens for long enough can be unnerving, boring or infuriating. This important phenomenon is known as projection, and how the process makes you feel is called the countertransference. If you cannot manage such feelings tickled up in you by the patient, you may wish to pursue him out of the consulting room and down the stairs, or indeed precede him. Or, more likely, you may pick up and react to more subtle personal feelings, for example that the patient may feel so hopeless that he makes you feel that he is not only beyond help, and moreover not worth helping, but that you are not much good either.

All this may be true. But, at least in theory, a training which helps you use psychodynamic models aims to help you respond on the level, rather than trying too hard or giving up too soon. Another example, perhaps closer to home medically speaking, relates to dependency by patients. Built into the traditional socio-cultural position of the doctor is the powerful notion of needing a strong figure with magical powers when faced with illness, pain and death or the fear of death. The need to help can influence one person's career choice as a doctor just as it may influence another's career choice as patient. Feelings of dependency and the counter-feeling of protectiveness may emerge in a clinical relationship in an unhelpful way, so that a patient's unconscious need to be looked after is matched by the doctor's unconscious need to look after others. The patient becomes chronic and the clinic overloaded.

In an ideal world, doctor and patient would have enough grasp of the emotional side of their mutual relationship to keep the relationship at an appropriate and helpful level – 'good enough', to adapt the psychoanalyst D.W. Winnicott's term for the parent who gets the balance about right between, among other things, overprotectiveness and underprotective-ness (Winnicott, 1974, 1991).

Principle 6

The moral neutrality of psychodynamic thinking has often caused misunder-standing. For example, the above account of the patient needing care and the doctor wishing to give it is not supposed to illustrate something good or bad, but just the way human beings operate. The dependent patient is no more 'bad' than the solicitous physician is 'good'. The psychoanalyst aspires to be non-judgmental. This is not because of perverted morality but an attempt to be a scientific observer of the therapist's and the patient's (or analysand's) feelings. When he disapproves of something the patient is doing (e.g. stealing, or drinking too much) he has to find a way of responding and guiding use-fully as a therapist, not as a policeman. However, this does not absolve the therapist from responsibilities as a citizen, as recent case law in the United States has shown, when it is necessary to warn a third person of a patient's malicious intent.

Principle 7

By the same token, you will understand a great deal about the psychody-namic model if you appreciate that in these vignettes we are not suggest-ing that there are 'out there' dreadfully dependent patients and overprotective clinicians, quite unlike sensible people like ourselves, but simply that tendencies toward such feelings are universal. The psychody-namic model suggests that such tendencies to incline in one direction (e.g. dependence, paranoia, sadness) or another (e.g. independence, trust, euphoria) are components of the psychology of all of us, and the points of balance shift and vary with different people in different circumstances and relationships at different times. Hence we can understand, if not agree with, the proclamation by Peter Simple's Dr Kiosk, in the *Daily Telegraph*, that 'we are all guilty'. It is when a particular frame of mind tends to predominate and endure regardless of the real circumstances that, if it is distressing or handicapping, it can become identified as a 'neurosis' (which is short for psychoneurosis) and it may then be amenable to one of the dynamic psychotherapies.

We could sum up the story so far by saying that the essence of the psychodynamic model is that things are not necessarily what they seem. The 'nice' person may 'invest' in niceness (initially) because they are busy managing paranoid feelings, or the 'happy' person may be coping well with sadness. These balancing acts are integral to normal human functioning and may or may not decompensate into something neurotic and disturbing.

Principle 8

Given this constant inner activity, we return again to the concept of the process being a dynamic one. Water may be at a constant level because of a balance between what flows in, what flows out and evaporation. Mental life has a constancy and rhythm, but the inner images, feelings and attitudes that constitute our moods and personalities are constantly being fed by perceptions from outside (traumatic, 'ordinary' and therapeutic) and no doubt by underground streams and fluctuating water tables too. But we digress into metaphors again.

Be all this as it may, such processes are not entirely random. The developing, maturing brain modulates itself, so that up to a point it 'hears what it wants to hear', and copes by keeping a balance between that which will fit in with existing beliefs and feelings and that which will upset the apple cart. Such defensive, adaptive processes, known as the mechanisms of defence, were part of classical Freudian theory, but developed further by Freud's daughter Anna (Freud, 1936). One example is rationalization. Earlier, we painted the picture of clinician and patient becoming thoroughly fed up (note the metaphor) with each other, indeed sick of each other. Nevertheless, it is possible to imagine not only the mutual courtesies with which the final appointment and the re-referral to someone else is arranged, but also the inner feelings on both sides that these practical steps are wholly positive, sensible and civilized; what a good doctor, patient, indeed clinic, and how reasonable we all are. And here is another twist: the re-referral may be necessary and the emotional 'background noise' authentic too. The dynamically fluctuating feelings operate at one level, rational decision making at another.

Another defence mechanism is denial, the insistence that something is not so when it very obviously is ('I am not angry!!'), and another is repression, when something is pushed firmly out of our awareness because it threatens psychological homeostasis. Projection has already been described. Reaction formation is a very nice example, when a forbidden drive that is taboo (for the individual, the community or usually both) is converted within into acceptable currency; thus the extreme solicitousness, albeit on a short fuse, of the irritable restaurateur – or doctor. The neurophysiological concept of the final common path is useful here (this describes the common nerve pathways at the end of a multiply complex system). Multiple twists, turns and interplay of feelings and ideas end up, for good or ill, in a particular pattern of thinking and behaviour, capable of being elicited by the social microclimate of the moment, or not.

Principle 9

These and other vastly complex processes are fomenting not only in inner homeostatic activity (which tends to protect from unmanageable pain or distress), but in an outer social process too. Thus the therapist and patient parting amicably in the above example may indeed be all right. The alternatives were (a) the therapist understanding and deciding to work through the 'countertransference', or (b) not understanding what was going on sufficiently to handle the situation properly and getting into a destructive fight with the patient. So to this picture of hidden depths within the individual we should add the hidden depths within the interaction, as one set of hidden depths communicates with the other.

(*Exercise*: 'I really must go,' says the long-staying guest, leaning back in the armchair; 'What a shame, must you really?' asks the hostess, leaping to her feet. Consider the layers of feeling in this social interaction.)

At an aesthetic level, it is intriguing to consider what artists and composers may have put into their work even centuries ago, and which now conveys something to the observer or listener, yet which neither creator nor appreciator could necessarily put into words. We mention this partly for diversionary amusement but also as a reminder that psychodynamic thinking is not considered as applicable only to the clinic, but to the whole of human life, not least to the arts.

Principle 10

We referred earlier to the need for creative skills if the ambiguous, contradictory and only half-perceived idea in our minds was to be grasped and communicated. Human beings are extraordinarily inventive, and the unique capacity for language is partly to do with the capacity to transform images and feelings into sounds and symbols that convey something of those images and feelings to others. We see this capacity for symbolism and non-verbal expression in some symptoms (page 58).

In the above 10 examples of fundamental principles of psychodynamic thinking we have used analogies from ordinary life as well as from the clinic; as said, psychodynamic psychology has much to say about the whole of mental life, normal, abnormal and borderline. However, the essence of psychodynamic psychotherapy is to recognize those processes, within the individual and reflected in the relationship, that are causing distress and handicap, and to try to change them. How to do so is beyond the scope and purpose of this book. However, we will not be daunted, and will try to outline in three sentences the essence of psychodynamic psychotherapy. First, the patient accepts at a rational, intellectual, cognitive level that he or she has a problem amenable to therapy based on conversation. This gradually changes to an emotionally laden relationship with the therapist within which feelings and attitudes about the self and the therapist can be identified, explored, and sorted into those worth keeping and those best let go; these are vivid, real and immediate, not hypothetical or recalled. (Hence the therapist's frequent reference to the 'here and now'.) The patient is thereby enabled, if all goes well, to become a different person within the therapeutic relationship, and the whole of the argument about whether or not psychodynamic psychotherapy 'works' rests upon whether or not he or she continues to be a different person outside it.

THE ESSENTIALS OF PSYCHODYNAMIC PSYCHOTHERAPY

- Intellectually, the patient expects change through talking with a therapist, even though change may not be wanted emotionally
- The 'ideas about feelings' that emerge in due course are not particularly useful. The feelings that matter therapeutically are the real feelings that emerge in the therapist–patient relationship
- If change for the better happens within this 'here and now' relationship, as it is called, it may be something the patients can take with them into future relationships

VARIATIONS ON THE THEME

Psychodynamic psychology is represented by an enormously rich literature and body of ideas which extend into many quite different types of clinical theory and practice, and outwards into the sciences, religion and the arts. For our limited purposes, to convey something of the variety, breadth and depth of the field, we will select fragments of different schools of thought.

Freud

From Sigmund Freud, we may draw attention to the crucial pleasure and pain principles, by which the organism is drawn towards that which gratifies and away from that which is less pleasurable and more painful. This reminds us of the amoeba (the one-celled organism that is similarly inclined to extending and growing towards pleasurable objects (e.g. food) and away from aversive ones (e.g. poison)). It is sometimes said that the first sign of life is irritability (Clark, 1947). It is also a reminder that first and foremost Freud was a biological thinker who believed that the neurophysiology of the future would support his theories (Sulloway, 1979).

Freudian theory is probably best known for its division of mental life into the ego, the superego and the id. We start with the id, in translation the 'it', a bundle of primitive instincts and impulses without direction or guidance beyond moving towards gratification on the pleasure–pain continuum. From this movement 'it' begins to learn something about external reality, and part of the id becomes differentiated into the self, and ultimately the self-conscious self, or ego. An important part of this reality is the social reality developed by other people, the expectations, rules and taboos in the family, the community and the culture in which the ego develops, and with which the ego has to come to terms. This adoption of 'the rules' by the developing individual makes up its superego, which, roughly speaking, is like his or her conscience. It largely picks up the rules, partly unconsciously, partly with mixed feelings (ambivalence again) from identification with parents or parent-figures by a process known as introjection (or 'taking on board', in the modern managerial parlance). As might well be imagined, there follows a great deal of struggling between the needs of the id, the dictates of the superego and the wishes of the ego, which by their psychodynamic interaction achieve a degree of homeostasis. If they do not, the individual or the community may suffer.

One fundamental task for the infant male to tackle, according to Freud, is how to cope with the discovery that another male, and indeed a big, strong one (daddy), also has an interest in the boy's own first love, his mother.

This could be dangerous, and represents the discovery of a love and sex that invited punishment, i.e. incest. This is the basic model for the distinguished Oedipal complex, the resolution of which (i.e. the coming to terms with) was regarded by Freud as a necessary challenge for boys. He was less clear about girls, about whose equivalent Electra complex less was said.

Freud is also known for his attention to dreams, the 'royal road to the unconscious'. His book, *The Interpretation of Dreams* (1954), is worth reading as a gripping work of literature, if nothing else. In brief, the psychodynamic model argues that dreams are charged with meaning. Physiological studies of sleep and dreaming confirm that dreaming, including the contents of dreams, has some function, but not particularly that which lends itself convincingly to Freudian interpretation. A reasonable view is that, as far as the brain is concerned, life goes on frenetically day and night rather as sketched on page xx, with events that include the random, the emotionally significant, and those which the individual can make useful stories from when awake, e.g. with his psychoanalyst.

A good, short account of Freudian ideas and those which derive from them is to be found in Brown (1961). An important reminder that Freud was trying to convey complex, subtle meanings that were not always adequately translated will be found in Bettelheim (1985). Two valuable and much larger works are by Wyss (1966) and Ellenberger (1970). Attachment theory is a more recent development which makes connections between psychoanalytic thinking, human relationships and our knowledge of animal behaviour (especially primates) and provides interesting models for symptom-formation. It is described on page xx. It is an example of the relatively new science of ethology, which is concerned with the evolution, purpose and meaning of behaviour.

Whatever we may make of Freud's ideas, they have become part of the culture (other models please note) and this says something interesting about the reciprocity between the evolution of mind and the development of language and literature (Steinberg, 2006). The literary critic, Bloom, writes of Freud as a great mythmaker, and 'no more a charlatan than the Socrates of Plato's *Symposium* . . . throwing Freud out will not get rid of him, because he is inside us. His mythology of the mind has survived his supposed science, and his metaphors are impossible to evade' (Bloom, 2002).

But we should give Freud the last word on metaphors and interpretations. 'Sometimes,' he is supposed to have said while puffing away, 'a cigar is just a cigar.'

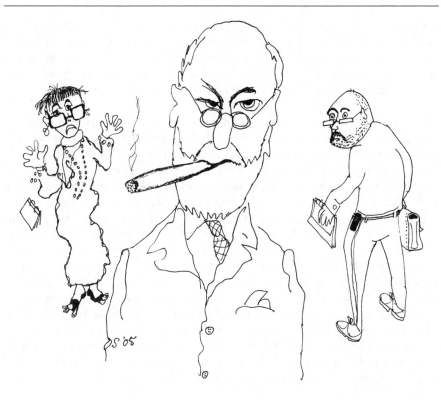

Jung

A whole school of psychodynamic psychology (known technically as analytic psychology) was developed by the Swiss psychiatrist C.G. Jung (1875–1961). If Freudian theory is in a sense psychobiological in its roots, Jungian theory is more based in cultural anthropology and mythology, although again with roots in social biology. Perhaps its most significant departure, or discovery, is the concept of the collective unconscious, and unconscious 'images' or potential images within it, known as the archetypes of the collective unconscious. These intriguing ideas have been widely misunderstood to refer to all sorts of alarming and provocative notions such as racial memories (inherited by some sort of discredited Lamarckian process) and mass telepathy, and to be fair to Jung's critics it may be said that some of his writing is contradictory and unclear on these and other themes.

However, it is well established by anthropologists and others that there are as many similarities as differences in the patterns of human behaviour and artistic and religious productions, even when there is no evidence of historical contact between various human groups. It is not far-fetched to suppose that the human imagination may have evolved within a developing human culture just as everything else about us has evolved (Steinberg, 2006), and that some inner fantasies and fancies, e.g. of gods, demons and big bad monsters, may be shared in common. Accounts of Jung from the biological perspective will be found in Stevens (2002), and developed in relation to dreaming in Stevens (1995).

To the uncommitted, but perhaps interested in Jung, the place for analytic psychology is really as a philosophical psychology that straddles anthropology, cultural history, spirituality and evolution more directly and comprehensively than the work of any of the other major figures in the history of psychodynamic ideas. It is intriguing, for example, that the concept of the archetype, one of Jung's most contentious formulations, and one which in the face of criticism he clarified as being *not* inherited ideas and images, but the inherited neuropsychological capacity for forming ideas and images, now seems to be consistent with many new developments in evolutionary psychology (Stevens, 2002) and with accounts of the neuroanatomy and neurophysiology of consciousness (Damasio, 1999; Steinberg, 2006). The exploratory and intuitive nature of much of Jung's writing, and even its ambiguities, lends itself to useful further interpretation and development. From the point of view of therapy, Jung's view of what is relevant in the human unconscious is not so much sexuality, but 'the fear of the (two-million-year-old) man crouching at the ford, as well as all the other fears and speculations born of man's experience through the ages' (Jung, 1935).

If Freudian psychotherapy tends towards the interpretation of unconscious material to do with sex, death and self-assertion, very much around the Oedipal theme and in the patient's own life, and with the patient doing most of the talking to a characteristically noncommittal analyst, then Jungian therapy tends towards the conversational, the universal rather than the reductionist, and to the individual's roots in his or her background and culture rather than in animal origins. Jungian therapists are also more inclined to use art techniques in therapy, e.g. painting and drawing. But, we emphasize, these are stereotypes, and there are as many types of practice as there are practitioners.

Adler

Alfred Adler (1870–1937), once the third great figure in the analytic trinity, has been relatively neglected in recent years in the UK, less so in North America. He founded individual psychology and we owe to him the concept of the inferiority complex and how disabilities can be compensated for in both neurotic and productive ways. His theories, and the practice deriving from them, are more reality-orientated and to do with setting goals, self-management and so on. He may return.

Klein

The ideas of Melanie Klein (1882–1960) can be baffling and to some have been infuriating, but one concept is particularly interesting and valuable and can show the way into a wider appreciation of her work. This is an elaboration of the notion of the ego's struggle (see page xx) in a period when the infant cannot distinguish between itself and the reality 'outside'. Feeling good (when gratified for example by food and warmth) and feeling bad (when these things are absent) are attributed (projected) as outside phenomena, i.e. as 'good objects' and 'bad objects'. The former are the objects of the infant's intense love, to be totally taken in, and the latter are the objects of hatred, to be destroyed or at least controlled. The primitive feelings developing at this stage 'in a world peopled by gods and devils' (Brown, 1961) was termed the paranoid position, and a very instructive position it is, if you allow that psychodynamic ideas about infants might throw light on political as well as clinical positions.

But there is more to this account. In due course the child makes a painful and formative discovery: that the object of its love, and of its hatred, are one and the same: the sometimes-gratifying and sometimes-non-gratifying mother. The child is still immature enough to believe in magic, that his love can preserve his mother and his hate can destroy her, and he is in a confused and ambivalent position. From this he can regress to the comforts of the paranoid position (where everything is easily classified good or bad, black or white), or try to make sense of his new discovery, which is a depressing experience (nothing's that simple; wait; be patient, put up with it; hear both sides; persevere) known as the depressive position. In Kleinian theory, and in therapy informed by its principles, the experience and acceptance of depression represents progress and a maturational step forwards, as indeed it can be in life outside therapy.

Klein described all this in terms of the mental life of the child in the first two or three months. It is easy for Klein's critics and proponents to become caught up on the argument (often, a blazing row) about whether anyone could know anything so specific about so young an infant, still less whether it can be of use, as Klein believed, in psychotherapy for children. And yet a look at human affairs in the newspapers or closer to home suggests that this model of infantile behaviour and its consequences has a heuristic value and a degree of face validity. As with Freud and Jung, the writings of Melanie Klein are still being sifted through, clarified and re-evaluated, and are very far from dead. They still create lively debate and their value is illustrated by a commendably clear and critical account by Hinshelwood (1994).

Psychodynamic theory is stronger on the general causes of human distress and the results of problems or breakdown in relationships than on the explanation of specific symptoms, which may be diverting and misleading. Thus in Kleinian terms the psychodynamic model provides a possible explanation for anger and depression when reality intrudes on an over-dependent relationship. The Freudian model can explain some patterns of anxiety and guilt when someone with problems in self-esteem and self-confidence feels they have over-asserted themselves in general, or in a particular relationship, and expect and fear retribution. In such psychodynamic explanations of symptoms there is the assumption that intense feelings belonging to childhood can be reactivated when someone is under pressure and, in emotional and perhaps behavioural terms too, he or she regresses.

ATTACHMENT THEORY

An interesting model for regression derives from attachment theory, really a set of models and theories developed by John Bowlby (Bowlby, 1969, 1973, 1980; and see Knox, 2003) which link psychodynamic concepts, parent–child behaviour and animal (especially primate) behaviour. The illustration below gives a simplified model of a dynamic interaction between a dependent child and a care-taking adult, with the child's proximity-seeking attachment behaviour (e.g. crying, 'attention-seeking', etc.) balanced by 'good enough' parenting or care-taking behaviour so that the child is neither neglected nor overprotected, and can therefore undertake the sort of exploratory behaviour that is expected in children and biologically necessary in human development. If the child's attachment behaviour does not trigger sufficient care-taking behaviour (because of a problem on either or both sides of the relationship) it tries, so the model goes, the behaviour that worked 'before', i.e. when the child was younger. Thus a plea, then nagging, then crying, all falling on deaf ears so to speak, might lead the child to regress to previous ways of eliciting a reaction, such as screaming, misbehaviour or complaining of stomach-ache or feeling sick.

The same model provides a descriptive explanation of the means by which experiences become incorporated in the developing personality (introjection again). The illustration on the previous page conveys events becoming incorporated as experience (or more likely set of experiences, and therefore assumptions about parenting), so that the child grows up with a tendency to expect the worst, feel anxious, not to trust, have a low self-esteem or to have somatic symptoms when anxious, and perhaps with problems in eventual parenting skills. Hence also behaviour within the family system, and perhaps amenable to family therapy (page xx), becomes part of the individual's own repertoire as an individual disorder needing individual or family treatment. This model indicates a more fundamental aspect of living systems: their circularity rather than linearity, their complexity, and their developmental nature (Steinberg, 2005) and represents aspects of systems theory.

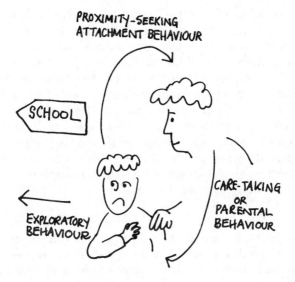

Model of a dynamic interaction between a dependent child
and a care-taking adult

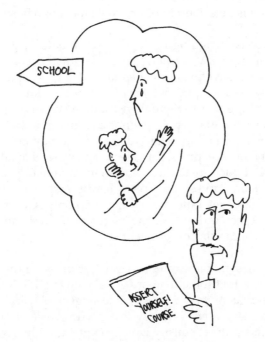

Incorporation of events as experience

There is little evidence of a single 'traumatic experience' being behind the development of neuroses and maladaptive personality traits. Children are relatively resilient. Rather it is the accumulation of such negative experiences in a persisting pattern of youthful problems and parental mishandling that establishes feelings and behaviours we later describe as psychiatric conditions. Attachment theory provides some illuminating models for this. Parkes (1969) provides similar socio-psychodynamic models. These demonstrate the similarities between the depressive symptoms of grief, the similar symptoms following amputation and other losses, and the actual behaviour of young humans and primates when separated from parents, with 'grieving' behaviour in the latter. Here biological observations tend to confirm the psychoanalytic metaphor of the 'search for a lost object'.

Hysteria (originally attributed to the uterus wandering about the body) remains a puzzle. It may be defined as the resort to symbolic problems when, for some reason, the direct expression of anxiety or distress is blocked. This may be due to immaturity, to cultural convention, to another aspect of neurotic personality structure (e.g. denial at all costs) or to the situation being extraordinarily difficult. In recent years, for example, many psychiatrists have begun to see hysterical behaviour such as simulated physical disability (e.g. paralysis, inability to swallow) in young people with a history of sexual abuse. Sometimes this takes the form of such chaotic thinking and behaviour that the condition is described as or mistaken for, a psychosis.

Anorexia nervosa is intriguing in this respect. Whatever its likely multiple bio-psychosocial origins, a psychodynamic formulation sometimes provides compelling reasons why the girl (incidentally, 10% of patients are male) does not want to grow up, and appears to have the uncanny knack of holding back her weight at just the point where menstruation ceases. Anxiety or depression may be associated with phobic symptoms such as a wish to escape from the scene or a fear of falling; again, the problem may be low self-esteem, shame or fear of failure, expressed as a fear of being seen to fall in public. The language is full of such metaphors – the fallen woman, 'collapse of stout party' in old cartoons, and so on. This is hardly surprising: the language of illness and the language of literature, from soap operas to real operas, come from the same source. And so does the language of psychoanalysis. But why does this surprise a certain sort of scientist?

This universality of symbolic expression can obscure as well as illuminate. The patient with a sense that something has gone wrong within him and of developing psychic incapacity may express his feelings in classical psychoanalytic terms. He might have a classical psychoanalytic problem, but the problem could be a disorder of the chemistry which maintains normal moods, or a neurodegenerative disorder. The patient who feels weak and dizzy and dreams of being caught undressed in the street may have a neurosis, a personality problem or anaemia. None of this invalidates the psychodynamic model for some patients, or for some aspects of some patients.

Mentalization

In recent years there has been great deal of interest in a phenomenon called mentalization. This is a very good example of something that cannot be properly expressed in any of the other models described in this book. Mentalization has been nicely summarized by my colleague Jeremy Holmes in a little section of the *British Journal of Psychiatry* called '100 words', in which whatever is being described cannot go over this word limit. Here is how he puts it:

> 'Mentalisation: 'mind-mindedness', the ability to see ourselves as others see us, and others as they see themselves; to appreciate that all human experience is filtered through the mind and therefore that all perceptions, desires and theories are necessarily provisional. Psychotherapy, whether cognitive or psychoanalytic, aims to enhance mentalisation skills and to identify situations in which mentalisation is impaired. Mentalisation and arousal are inimical – stress interferes with the ability to mentalise effectively. Stressed non-mentalising psychiatrists and their patients, especially those with borderline personality disorder, are less likely to make good decisions than their mentalising counterparts. Training helps overcome this.'
>
> (Holmes, 2008)

Mentalization has been picked up by the cognitive-behavioural model but it really belongs with the psychodynamic one. It is not just a simple issue of identifying dysfunctional thoughts, but appreciating how they arise and influence behaviour.

THE EVOLUTIONARY MODEL

We have already mentioned the calumny on the part of many of the detractors of psychodynamic theory that it has remained firmly stuck to the analyst's couch for the last hundred years or so. On the contrary, one of the most interesting recent developments in conceptual thinking owes much to the thinking of psychodynamic theorists who have shown some consistencies between aspects of psychoanalytic theory, evolution and animal sociobiology (e.g. Bowlby, 1969, 1973, 1980; Parkes, 1969; Stevens, 2002; Stevens and Price, 1996). The essence of this new ethological thinking is that many psychiatric problems can be understood as patterns of thinking and behaviour which were adaptive in the very early, primitive conditions of the human race, and being crucial for survival have remained part of our repertoire even though generally redundant. For example it is self-evident that anxiety is necessary for survival, and yet in certain people in certain circumstances can be precipitated as an excessive, inappropriate and disabling state. Thus a state of anxiety and suspiciousness bordering on paranoia might be literally life-saving on a dark night if one strayed too far towards the trees from one's cave, but could be a nuisance if the same feeling pattern was precipitated towards one's surroundings in a pleasant suburb. Although, come to think of it, maybe not.

An interesting case has been made by Stevens and Price (1996) that the capacity to be depressed could have evolved as an adaptive way of accepting defeat when deposed in a social hierarchy, thus enabling the rank order to be maintained rather than disintegrating into anarchy. Correspondingly, the restless, agitated distress associated with grief, mentioned on page xx, could serve both to raise the chances of finding again a lost relative, or of recruiting help if the loss proves permanent. Schizophrenic spectrum disorders can be so destructive that, coupled with the relatively lower fertility of people with these conditions, it is a surprise that the condition has survived at all. However, first, it is likely to be represented genetically by a number of different genetic predispositions, and, intriguingly, there is evidence that genetically related people without the illness may include a higher than expected incidence of individuals with creative or religious leanings. How might that be useful in evolutionary terms? Stevens and Price (1996) have argued that the emergence of charismatic leaders who convince themselves and many others of a new future and a promised land, characteristically associated with much new ritual and the identification of the new grouping as the 'in group', may have enabled new groups and tribes to form when previous groups broke down or split. This has resulted in much murder and mayhem in the modern world, but in the past would have helped preserve the species, heaven help us.

On which note we may need to warn the enlightened reader that mentioning evolutionary theory can cause as much alarm and opposition in some social science circles as it does among fundamentalists who believe in divine creation. Even among social scientists, suggestions that we may be influenced by our territorially minded primate ancestors can produce much primitive, angry tooth and buttock baring; see, for example, the accounts in Rose and Rose (2000) and Segerstråle (2000).

PRACTICAL APPLICATIONS

The content and implications of psychodynamic theory tend to be protean, as well they might, considering that it comprises a highly variegated but universal model for human mental life, and involves biology, social science, anthropology, religion and the arts in its broad philosophy. Not surprisingly, you could derive many different areas of work and forms of practice from a field which has had so many contributions over the past hundred years.

Individual psychoanalysis still stands, or lies, with the analysands going five times a week for a couple of years for their 'first' analysis, although we understand a second analysis can be as *de rigueur* as a farmhouse in France. The indications for psychoanalysis as treatment are not discussed here, but from the point of view of professional training it is understandable that a training analysis is appropriate for psychotherapists who intend to practise psychoanalysis or psychoanalytic psychotherapy, as a necessary aid to clear thinking and appropriate responses when the projections begin to fly.

This is a reminder (from the ever-helpful unconscious) that we forgot all about Freudian slips. There was a nice example during the 1992 Conservative Party Conference when a senior UK politician was being interviewed about what Margaret Thatcher was like to work with. He referred to blazing rows 'when she would hit the fan'.* However, he did not get the saying quite right. Like dreams, Freudian slips may be guided by significant feelings, or be entirely random, or due to other influences (e.g. the proximity of certain keys on the typewriter keyboard) or by a combination of these things.

The psychodynamic model includes pychodynamic psychotherapy as systematic psychotherapy guided by psychodynamic principles, in which the practitioner may be thoroughly trained or hardly trained at all, and may be practically indistinguishable from psychoanalysis at one end of the spectrum, to hardly recognizable at all as psychotherapy at the other. The field is very variable; but within it there is much highly skilled, dedicated work of the highest integrity.

Precisely the same is true of a vast range of creative, or 'humanistic' and 'progressive' psychotherapies, and those with a special focus such as marital relationships and sex. Here psychotherapy and counselling blur into each other, although one might define the former as being concerned with fundamental change in feelings and the latter more to do with advice, practical management and self-management.

Drama therapy and *art therapy* are forms of therapy where activity, such as acting roles or expressing feelings in paint and other art work, take precedence

---

*Readers who do not understand the joke are invited to apply to the author for an explanation.

over words in establishing the therapeutic relationship and representing feelings. For children, play therapy is a technique with similarities to this.

It may be supposed that such techniques are particularly useful where the patient is less articulate; on the contrary, a patient with highly developed verbal skills may deal with feelings in too intellectual a way, and the techniques of art and drama can then usefully bypass overactive 'higher centres'. Jennings (1983) provides an excellent overview of the creative therapies in very practical terms, and Thomson (1989) an outstanding short guide to the principles of art therapy.

Psychodynamic therapy has long concerned itself with personality problems, and has stuck with trying to help people with such difficulties even when other parts of psychiatry had doubts whether such problems should be treated by mental health services at all. Integrated care in a psychodynamic framework has now been shown to be of considerable value in at least one group, those with the complex and diffuse personality organization known as borderline personality disorder (Bateman and Fonagy, 1999, 2004).

Family therapy, which itself contains many schools of thought and practice, is similarly concerned with actions more than words. The family therapies have more or less in common the principle that what is inferred in the 'one-to-one' or dyadic therapeutic session can be seen played out before the eyes of all concerned in family therapy. For example, if a boy forms a teasing alliance with his mother and excludes the father, who gets ever angrier, the family therapist might intervene with comments or actions. The therapist might invite the mother to move her position to where she can see her husband's reaction, and ask the father if he is happy with his son leaning his head on his mother's shoulder, and does he want to ask him to move? Family therapy may broadly follow group analytic lines (i.e. psychoanalytic theory as applied to groups) or systemic theory, with many variations.

The latter is an interesting model based on systems theory (see page xx) rather than psychoanalytic theory; it represents a social rather than psychological dynamic, in that the system (e.g. a family group) reaches a particular state of homeostasis in which (for example) various roles become fixed, e.g. the misbehaving adolescent, the 'good' but depressed big sister, the workaholic husband and the alcoholic wife. The presenting symptom, or in family therapy parlance the identified patient, may be the naughty boy, but he may in some respects be the 'healthiest' family member, challenging the family's stability (unconsciously) to draw attention to a range of (denied) problems. The small boat with several people in it is quite a good model to understand family therapy; if one person changes position everyone else has to move, some more than others, to achieve stability again. In the process the presenting problems can diminish and others be identified. Family therapy has an enormous number of good introductory books, all very different. One, by Robin Skynner and John Cleese (1984), deals with individual and family dynamics. Gorrell Barnes (1994) and Bloch and Harari (2000) provide helpful reviews. Another approach to handling the roles and myths involved in anomalous relationships is to consider the stories or 'scripts' being followed, albeit unconsciously, as in *narrative therapy* (White and Epston, 1990), while Steinberg (2000) has described similar approaches in letter-writing both to patients and professionals.

In family therapy we are another step away from traditional psychodynamic theory and closer to group and social theory, with their counterparts not only in small group therapies (with some overlap with family therapy), but in the understanding of large groups too, including very large groups and groupings in organizations such as hospitals and other institutions (Kreeger, 1975; Skynner, 1989). Here, on the outer edge of the psychodynamic universe, we enter another world, one pioneered by the Tavistock Institute in London, where the dynamics of the interaction not only between people and groups but between departments, agencies and professions have been explored (e.g. Caplan, 1970; Steinberg, 1989, 2005; Trist and Murray, 1990). At this point we have gone full circle and are looking at models for social systems which foster, or fail to foster, individual development.

CONCLUSION

What is most intriguing about psychodynamic theory is not only that it is a rich mixture of the implausible and the commonsensical, the banal and the brilliant, but that many sensible people disagree over which is which. Taken overall, the special gift to the clinician of the psychodynamic model is not to help make oversimplified and ultimately wrong assumptions about psychiatric disorders and other aspects of feelings and behaviour, but to appreciate the rich complexity of people's lives, our development and, ultimately, our evolution. When all the other models in this book are examined it is the psychodynamic one that is the most explanatory and revealing. It is against this biological and biographical background that the pain in the neck, or indeed in the backside, can be more fully understood; it is a long way from the simplistic hydraulic model that made the approach so much the butt of scornful critics who dismissed it as outmoded.

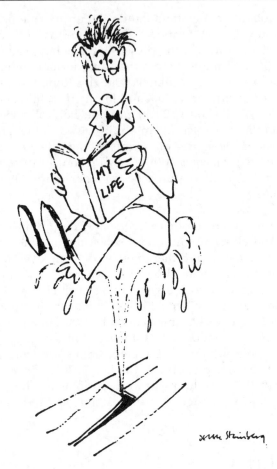

'. . . it is a long way from the simplistic hydraulic model'

REFERENCES

Bateman, A. and Fonagy, P. (1999) Effectiveness of partial hospitalization in the treatment of borderline personality disorder: a randomized controlled trial. *American Journal of Psychiatry*, **156**, 1563–1569.

Bateman, A. and Fonagy, P. (2004) *Psychotherapy for Borderline Personality Disorder: Mentalization Based Treatment*. Oxford University Press, Oxford.

Bettelheim, B. (1985) *Freud and Man's Soul*. Fontana, London.

Bloch, S. and Harari, E. (2000) Family therapy. In: M. Gelder, J. Lopez-Ibor and N. Andreasen (eds), *The New Oxford Textbook of Psychiatry*, pp. 1472–1483. Oxford University Press, Oxford.

Bloom, H. (2002) *Genius*. Fourth Estate: London.

Bowlby, J. (1969) *Attachment and Loss*. Volume 1: *Attachment*. Hogarth Press, London.

Bowlby, J. (1973) *Attachment and Loss*. Volume 2: *Separation: Anxiety and Anger*. Hogarth Press, London.

Bowlby, J. (1980) *Attachment and Loss*. Volume 3: *Loss*. Hogarth Press, London.
Brown, J.A.C. (1961) *Freud and the Post-Freudians*. Penguin Books, Harmondsworth.
Caplan, G. (1970) *The Theory and Practice of Mental Health Consultation*. Tavistock, London.
Clark, Le Gros (1947) *The Tissues of the Body*. Cambridge University Press, Cambridge.
Damasio, A. (1999) *The Feeling of What Happens: Body, Emotion and the Making of Consciousness*. Heinemann, London.
Ellenberger, H.F. (1970) *The Discovery of the Unconscious*. Allen Lane, London.
Evans, P. (1972) Henri Ey's concepts of the organisation of consciousness and its disorganisation: an extension of Jacksonian theory. *Brain*, **95**, 2, 413–420.
Freud, A. (1936) *The Ego and the Mechanisms of Defence*. Hogarth Press, London.
Freud, S. (1954) *The Interpretation of Dreams*, trans. J. Strachey. George Allen and Unwin, London.
Gorrell Barnes, G. (1994) Family therapy. In: M. Rutter, E. Taylor and L. Hersov (eds), *Child Psychiatry: Modern Approaches*, 3rd edn, pp. 946–967. Blackwell Science, Oxford.
Hinshelwood, R.D. (1994) *Clinical Klein*. Free Association Books, London.
Holmes, J. (2008) Mentalisation: a key skill for psychiatrists and their patients – in 100 words. *British Journal of Psychiatry*, **193**, 125.
Jennings, S. (1983) *Creative Therapy*. Kemble Press, Banbury.
Jung, C.G. (1935) *Analytical Psychology: Its Theory and Practice*. Tavistock Lectures: in *Collected Works*, Volume 18. Routledge & Kegan Paul, London.
Knox, J. (2003) *Archetype, Attachment, Analysis*. Brunner-Routledge, London.
Kreeger, L. (1975) *The Large Group*. Constable, London.
Parkes, C.M. (1969) Separation anxiety: an aspect of the search for a lost object. In: M.H. Lader (ed.) *Studies of Anxiety*. Royal Medico-Psychological Association, London.
Rose, H. and Rose, S. (eds) (2000) *Alas, Poor Darwin. Arguments against Evolutionary Psychology*. Radcliffe Publishing, Abingdon.
Segerstråle, U. (2000) *Defenders of the Truth: The Sociobiology Debate*. Oxford University Press, Oxford.
Skynner, R. (1989) In: J. Schlapobersky (ed.) *Institutes and How to Survive Them*. Methuen, London.
Skynner, R. and Cleese, J. (1984) *Families and How to Survive Them*. Methuen, London.
Steinberg, D. (1989) *Interprofessional Consultation. Innovation and Imagination in Working Relationships*. Blackwell Scientific, Oxford.
Steinberg, D. (2000) *Letters from the Clinic. Letter Writing in Clinical Practice for Mental Health Professionals*. Brunner-Routledge, London.
Steinberg, D. (2005) *Complexity in Healthcare and the Language of Consultation: Exploring the Other Side of Medicine*. Radcliffe Publishing, Abingdon.
Steinberg, D. (2006) *Consciousness Reconnected: Missing Links between Neuroscience, Depth Psychology and the Arts*. Radcliffe Publishing, Abingdon.
Stevens, A. (1995) *Private Myths. Dreams and Dreaming*. Hamish Hamilton, London.
Stevens, A. (2002) *Archetypes Revisited*. Brunner-Routledge, London.
Stevens, A. and Price, J. (1996) *Evolutionary Psychiatry*. Routledge, London.
Sulloway, F.J. (1979) *Freud: Biologist of the Mind*. André Deutsch, London.
Thomson, M. (1989) *On Art and Therapy*. Virago, London.
Trist, E. and Murray, H. (eds) (1990) *The Social Engagement of Social Science*. A Tavistock Anthology. Volume 1: *The Socio-psychological Perspective*. Free Association Books, London.
White, M. and Epston, D. (1990) *Narrative Means to Therapeutic Ends*. W.W. Norton, London.

Wilson, P. (1986) Individual psychotherapy in a residential setting. In: D. Steinberg (ed.) *The Adolescent Unit*. Wiley, Chichester.

Winnicott, D.W. (1974) *Playing and Reality*. Penguin, Harmondsworth.

Winnicott, D.W. (1991) *Human Nature*. Free Association Books, London.

Wyss, D. (1966) *Depth Psychology: A Critical History*. George Allen and Unwin, London.

$\boxed{4}$

THE COGNITIVE-
BEHAVIOURAL MODEL

'Freudian theory regards neurotic symptoms as "the visible upshot of unconscious causes". Learning theory does not postulate any such "unconscious" causes, but regards neurotic symptoms as simply learned habits; there is no neurosis underlying the symptom but merely the symptom itself. Get rid of the symptom and you have eliminated the neurosis'.

H.J. Eysenck, 1965

'And thus the native hue of resolution
Is sicklied o'er with the pale cast of thought
And enterprises of great pith and moment
In this regard, their currents turn awry
And lose the name of action'

William Shakespeare, Hamlet

DIFFERENCES FROM OTHER MODELS

In the second and third editions of this book we separated cognitive and behavioural models but it is now clear that they belong together. It is also equally clear that this model is a more generic one involving structured collaborative approaches to both thinking and emotions. So the student should not get too hung up over the cognitive-behavioural aspects; a range of other approaches, including schema-focused therapy, social skills training, many education training methods, and other applications of learning theory are all part of the model. There is even one treatment, cognitive analytical therapy, that crosses over to the psychodynamic model combines both approaches (Ryle, 1997). The cognitive-behavioural model adopts a fundamentally different approach from the biological, psychodynamic and social models vying for your attention elsewhere in this book. This is seen most starkly in their respective views of mental symptoms.

Models for Mental Disorder: Conceptual Models in Psychiatry, Fifth Edition. Peter Tyrer.
© 2013 John Wiley & Sons, Ltd. Published 2013 by John Wiley & Sons, Ltd.

The psychodynamic psychotherapist regards patients' symptoms as presenting features that obscure and mislead rather than edify or explain. Symptoms are seen not just as the tip of an iceberg but as a decoy, an iceberg that is separated completely from its complete submerged partner and which is set up deliberately to confuse. If the symptoms are treated directly they will only reappear in another form (symptom substitution) and so they should be regarded as clues to the underlying problem but having no real substance. The biological psychiatrist differs in finding symptoms useful but only as the building blocks of disease entities that can help in identification. Adherents to the social model see symptoms as culturally determined reactions to social forces that have no special significance in themselves apart from serving a purpose as markers of illness behaviour.

The cognitive-behavioural model concentrates on symptoms and thinking as the core of mental disorder. 'Get rid of the symptom and you have eliminated the neurosis' is indeed the message of the model, but it does not just apply to 'neurosis', now largely subsumed into a range of anxiety and depressive disorders in our new classifications, but to the whole of mental illness. By concentrating on the way in which symptoms and behaviour are formed, developed and changed, the model explains much more about mental illness than the other models and has a much better explanatory base; it can illustrate how mental illness can both develop and be resolved by direct empirical evidence. Indeed, the evidence base for the effectiveness of cognitive behaviour therapy exceeds that for all other treatments and has the great advantage of having very few adverse effects.

HOW THE COGNITIVE-BEHAVIOURAL MODEL DEVELOPED

Historically the behavioural component of this model was introduced first and achieved prominence with the work of Pavlov in the Soviet Union and Skinner In the United States, who developed the basics of learning theory and the origins of maladaptive behaviour. They were also influenced by the work of John B. Watson, an American psychologist from Johns Hopkins University who first developed the notion of behaviourism (or behaviorism in US English) after becoming enthused with the work of Pavlov and his experimental animals. Watson was concerned that the study of behaviour was regarded as a means of helping to understand consciousness, introspection, motivation and higher nervous processes (particularly in psychoanalysis), but not as a discipline in its own right. He felt that behaviourism was a well-demarcated scientific subject that could stand on its own with other subjects without the need to invoke consciousness or indeed any of the other psychologies that were prominent at the time. So he wrote, in words that would have been surprisingly apposite many years later:

> 'Psychology, as the behaviorist views it, is a purely objective, experimental branch of natural science which needs introspection as little as do the sciences of chemistry and physics. It is granted that the behavior of animals can be investigated without appeal to consciousness. Heretofore the viewpoint has been that such data have value only in so far as they can be interpreted by analogy in terms of consciousness. The position is taken here that the behavior of man and the behavior of animals must be considered on the same plane; as being equally essential to a general understanding of behavior. It can dispense with consciousness in a psychological sense.'
>
> (Watson, 1913)

Thus psychologists were reassured that their work had general value; they should not feel that they were carrying out minor studies that might help those working on the higher orders of mental activity; they were scientists pursuing knowledge in its own right and had the data to develop and understand it without recourse to any other discipline. This had a major influence on studies of human behaviour and the learning process involved in its development. Learning goes on all the time but is usually appropriate,

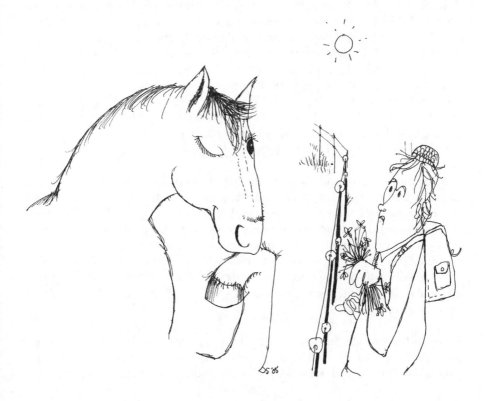

responsive to situations and therefore adaptive. The first time we see an electric fence keeping horses in a field we may touch it inadvertently. The electric shock we receive is unpleasant so we take care to avoid further contact. We have acquired new learning very quickly and will be careful when we come across an electric fence again. The same learning process is carried out on the other side of the electric fence by the horses; there is no fundamental difference in the acquisition of this knowledge between the two species.

Learning theory is a psychological science that has an excellent pedigree. Two forms of conditioning are responsible for the formation of most maladaptive behaviour, classical and operant conditioning. Classical conditioning refers to learning that takes place when a neutral stimulus becomes associated with a previously unrelated sequence of a stimulus and response. The stimulus and response are directly linked; one follows from the other in the behavioural model without any complicated processes intervening. This omission of mental processes makes the psychotherapist profoundly uncomfortable, because such a notion deprives him of his bread and butter and would convert psychoanalysis into boring reflexology.

But the simple facts support the model. Classical conditioning was first described by Pavlov, in a celebrated series of experiments with dogs, first carried out in the study of salivation. It is worthwhile repeating this in some detail, even though classical conditioning is not often used in current treatment. Dogs (and other mammals – this includes us as well) salivate when eating. Having a plentiful supply of saliva helps in chewing food and also aids digestion as saliva contains enzymes which break down some of the food. Salivation normally starts when the dog smells the food so that by the time the first mouthful is taken there is saliva already secreted. All this makes good physiological sense and was known many years before Pavlov's experiments. The stimulus of food is followed by the response of salivation.

Pavlov introduced measurement to this phenomenon by cannulating the salivary ducts of the dogs so that the exact quantity of saliva could be recorded. He was then able to see if other stimuli altered salivary flow. By itself, the sound of a bell had no effect on salivary flow. But if the bell was sounded at or about the same time food was presented to the dog, after several trials the sound of the bell alone was enough to produce a copious flow of saliva. In other words, the neutral stimulus of the bell ringing had become linked to the stimulus (food)–response (salivation) and thereby had become a conditional stimulus.

Now on the surface this experiment does not appear to be a breakthrough. The results probably could be predicted correctly by many who had no pretensions to special knowledge in the biological sciences. Indeed, the animal-lover Bernard Shaw (1932), speaking as usual through the mouths of his characters, says of this experiment,*

'Why didn't you ask me? I could have told you in 25 seconds without hurting those poor dogs.'

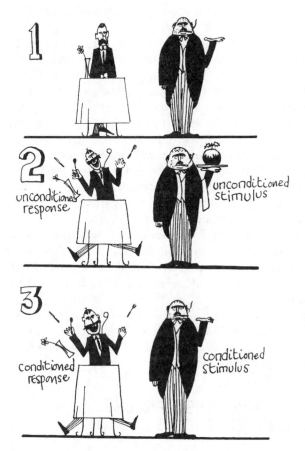

'The stimulus of food is followed by the response of salivation'

Where Pavlov broke entirely new ground was in his detailed examination of the factors that increase (positively reinforce) or reduce (negatively reinforce and, ultimately, extinguish) the conditioned response. The greater the frequency and the closer the bell and food were presented together in time, the stronger was the conditioning. Further experiments showed that when the dogs were put under stress their conditioned responses became disturbed. For

---

* In *The Adventures of the Black Girl in Her Search for God.*

example, a dog that had been conditioned to salivate in response to a circle but not to an ellipse displayed increasing signs of agitation when the ellipse was changed gradually until it was almost circular. Anxiety and agitation inhibit salivation and even when the dog was capable of making the correct choice salivary flow was not as great as formerly. Eventually Pavlov was able to produce a comprehensive physiological theory of abnormal behaviour based entirely on his experiments with classical conditioning (Pavlov, 1927, 1941).

Operant conditioning differs from classical conditioning in that behaviour determines conditioning, not the stimulus. The psychologist B.F. Skinner was the father of operant conditioning (Skinner, 1972) and the Skinner box, which he invented, is one of the best methods of illustrating it in practice. A Skinner box consists of a closed box with one or more buttons, levers or switches which can be operated by an animal placed in the box. If a hungry pigeon is put in the box it will not at first have any stimulus – response patterns to reinforce so conditioning will not occur. However, in the course of exploring its new environment it is likely to peck at one of the buttons at the side of the box. If this is the correct button a small amount of food will be delivered into the box from a hopper outside. After gobbling this up the pigeon wants more. He does not know how the food arrived but before long he links the pecking of the button with the arrival of food. Once this is learnt the button will be pecked repeatedly until his appetite is satisfied. In this case positive reinforcement of the conditioned response (pecking the button) will be increased by the continual supply of food and extinguished by ceasing to provide food when the button is pecked. Unlike classical conditioning, which depends on the experimenter manipulating a neutral stimulus so that it becomes a conditioned one, operant conditioning is determined by the animal's own behaviour. If the pigeon shows no exploratory behaviour when it is put in the Skinner box it will not be conditioned.

MOVING BEHAVIOURISM FROM THE LABORATORY TO THE CLINIC

These experiments of Skinner and Pavlov are now very well known, but they have been described in detail because they emphasize two important points. First, the behavioural model is based on scientific experiment and involves measurement that can be replicated (unlike many components of the psychodynamic model); secondly, the learning theory underpinning it is also based on replicable experiment. Behaviourism allows the scientist to observe, manipulate by experiment and develop testable theories from the results.

As learning theory applies to humankind as well as animals the same principles also apply. Thus, in a replication of Pavlov's work, Watson and Rayner

(1920) (yes the same Watson who introduced behaviourism) presented a young boy with a tame white rat at the same time as sounding a loud noise. The young boy was frightened by the loud noise and, not surprisingly, came to associate this with the presence of the rat. He therefore became frightened of the rat. Such fear is normally regarded as unreasonable and such irrational fears are called phobias. The boy's phobia of white rats soon developed to a phobia of all furry animals, a phenomenon called 'generalization' by the behaviourists.

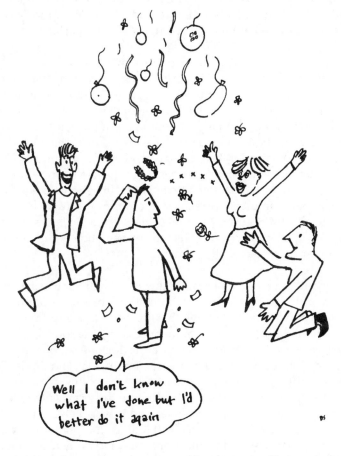

'... operant conditioning is determined by the animal's own behaviour'

Normally when a response is not reinforced it is extinguished, but a phobia initiated in this way tends to persist. This is because people with phobias usually deal with their fears by a special form of behaviour (avoidance) that prevents exposure to the phobic stimulus. Although this appears to work in the short term (i.e. it reduces the fear), in the longer term it tends to reinforce it. This clearly makes sense. Each time you avoid a situation because you think it will make you anxious the fear you attach to this situation will increase *as there is no way of demonstrating to you that the situation is harmless.*

This is how the pattern of maladaptive responses becomes established. The boy in Watson's experiment was conditioned to fear rats under the circumstances of the experiment. He then tended to avoid rats so the fear was reinforced. Each time subsequently he is exposed to furry animals he feels frightened and runs away (conditioned avoidance response) so he never gets a chance to realize that laboratory-bred rats are really harmless.

To restore a normal response the maladaptive one has to be replaced with an adaptive pattern of behaviour. This can be done by removing the fear response gradually, through imagining or being exposed to different, carefully graded levels of the phobic stimulus while relaxed (systematic desensitization), or dramatically, by preventing avoidance (flooding or 'implosion'). Desensitization and flooding can also be combined in gradual exposure to the phobic stimulus. Better response is obtained if the patient carries out the treatment programme in real life rather than imagination (exposure *in vivo*). In many ways desensitization is the reverse of acquisition of the phobia. Images or actual representations of the phobic stimuli are presented in order from a furry toy, to a rabbit and finally to a live rat during deep relaxation. Once the lowest phase in the hierarchy is completed successfully (i.e. the presentation of the toy evokes no fear), the next stage is taken in the same way.

These treatments, all based on learning theory, were first described by Wolpe (1958) who concluded that 'reciprocal inhibition' was the important ingredient. Phobic fear was inhibited by the presence of relaxation elsewhere. Reciprocal inhibition is now seldom mentioned in relationship to desensitization. It derives from neurology, as in order for one set of muscles in the body to contract the opposing set of muscles has to relax and this is automatically achieved by the nervous system. However, this is an analogy of behaviour therapy rather than an equivalent, so the term is now rarely used. It is better to conclude that the maladaptive phobic behaviour is counter-conditioned by the desensitization. In flooding, the phobic person is put in the situation that makes him most anxious, and is then prevented from escaping from it. The principle of treatment is explained in advance; escape from the fear only reinforces the idea that the situation is dangerous. If escape is prevented the person's level of anxiety goes up at first but falls later as he realizes that the terrible consequences he fears do not in fact happen. In exposure therapy the subject is encouraged to tackle the fears gradually. Instead of being flung in at the deep end he tests the water gradually, moving steadily down towards the deeper levels, extinguishing his anxiety as he goes. Of course it is important for the therapist to reinforce the idea that the phobia is unjustified and make sure that there is nothing in the experimental situation that might support or replace the fears with new ones.

An excellent example of how not to desensitize a phobia of rats is described in the last pages of George Orwell's (1949) celebrated novel, *1984*, in which the hero, Winston Smith, is 'cleansed' of all his heretical ideas by going to 'Room 101', a dreadful place where each person's special fears are exploited by techniques that have long been known by the name of brainwashing. Winston has a specific phobia of rats and this is reinforced by the inquisition of 'Room 101' before a solution is offered by clever counterconditioning. He comes to understand that all his fears can be healed by forgetting his past notions and believing that the head of state, Big Brother, is the fount of truth and knowledge. When he says simply 'I love Big Brother' his counter-conditioning is complete. (Readers in the UK will note that 'Big Brother' and 'Room 101' are now such unmissable television programmes for so many that perhaps we have all become counter-conditioned.)

INTRODUCTION OF THE COGNITIVE COMPONENT

Behaviourism achieved a great deal between 1913 and 1960 but was a little constricting. Skinner's verdict that there was no such thing as 'mind' as 'all behaviour was rationally controlled by operant conditioning' seemed to miss out some very important precursors of behaviour, particularly the process of thinking. The cognitive component of the cognitive-behavioural model developed later, single-handedly at first, through the work of Aaron Tim Beck, preceded by Albert Ellis, who introduced rational emotive therapy as a precursor of the cognitive-behavioural model (Ellis, 1962) but which has now also embraced the behavioural component (Ellis, 1995). Beck was trained as a psychoanalyst but became disenchanted with the psychodynamic model because it seemed unnecessarily slow and not focused on change. When asked to analyse depressed patients' dreams – a classical psychodynamic approach to detect underlying hidden conflict – Freud's 'royal road to the unconscious' – Beck expected to find that depressed patients would be full of angry ferment and torment as predicted by analytic theory.

In fact, he found less evidence of hostility than in patients who were not depressed. What he did notice, much more strongly, was that depressed patients had very negative views of their worth, their relationships and their achievements that were clearly not based on fact, and that these too were reflected in their dreams. He then made the great leap in thinking from regarding these negative views as 'symptoms occurring as a consequence of depression' to seeing them as 'cognitive distortions engendering depression', and a new approach was born (Beck, 2006). By examining each of these cognitive distortions or errors in thinking he was able to guide the patients back to their former ways of thinking and so relieve the depressive symptoms. Because this treatment was often tested by behavioural experiments it became known as cognitive-behavioural therapy, often abbreviated to CBT.

Although the initial work with CBT was in sufferers from depression and anxiety (Beck, 1976; Beck et al., 1985; Blackburn and Davidson, 1995) it has now been extended to cover a very large part of psychiatry, including the treatment of schizophrenia and bipolar disorder (Kingdon and Turkington, 1993; Perry et al., 1999). The basic tenets of the model are simple: errors in thinking and their effect on behaviour are responsible for the generation, maintenance and perpetuation of mental illness. Thus René Descartes' famous aphorism 'Cogito ergo sum' (I think, therefore I am) could be tickled a little into 'Cogito perperam ergo insanio' (I think wrongly, therefore I am mentally ill), to describe the cognitive-behavioural model.

I was lucky enough to be present at a celebratory dinner hosted by the Association for Research into Personality Disorders (ARPD) for Tim Beck in 2006. In response to his talk I gave a vote of thanks in a Lancashire accent (the county of my birth). Tim had not come across the tendency of people from Lancashire to talk in plain but simple verse, but as his talk summarized how cognitive therapy began I had the opportunity to translate it into 'Lanky speak'. The following is my (slightly edited) summary that I would like to think is a helpful guide to this form of therapy (and a poke at the psychodynamic model):

The folks said – polite-like – just for me
"You must go to the ARPD"
I said "I can't" but were held in check
"You've got no choice, 'cos we've got Tim Beck"
"Ee, ee," I said, "p'raps I don't mind
Entertainment of a different kind"
Tim detailed to us in proper order
All his personality disorder
He said, "listen well, 'cos there's more than one"
And that really got me thinking on
Severe PD means total paralysis
Then he told us why – "psychoanalysis,
It doesn't worry when it gets stuck
It just rumbles on and makes it up"
We all felt sorry for disordered Tim
He barely knew what had happened to him
We could see his mind were wracked by torsion
Then the answer came, "cognitive distortion"

And that, my friends, is the history
Of what – till now's – been a mystery
We've been exposed to the ultimate verity
The real start of cognitive behaviour therapy'

CENTRAL TENETS OF THE COGNITIVE-BEHAVIOURAL MODEL

- People's view of their world is determined by their thinking (cognition)
- Cognition influences symptoms, behaviour, emotion and attitudes and, thereby, the main features of mental illness
- The persistence of mental illness is a consequence of continuing errors in thinking and maladaptive behaviour that become reinforcing
- Significant change in mental disorder is always associated with significant change in cognition and behaviour

---

TESTING THE MODEL

The central tenets of the cognitive-behavioural model are straightforward. Thinking and behaviour are the engines at the centre of our being and help to make the decisions that determine our destinies and which, under normal circumstances, keep us well. At first sight the notion of cognition as a primary operator in this model seems to be curious. Are the proponents of the cognitive model suggesting the mental disorder is 'all in the mind'? Surely thinking becomes disordered as a consequence of illness; can it really be the primary cause? And how do we know we are influencing cognition when we can only measure behaviour?

To answer these questions let us take a common superstition of childhood, that of touching a lamp-post before crossing the road. There are many childhood superstitions of this nature, including linking actions to numbers or days (e.g. only having a bath on a Thursday), walking on the 'squares' of pavements, not on the 'lines' separating them, or checking things and counting to a certain number on your fingers before undertaking an important task (e.g. running in a school race). In the case of touching the lamp-post before crossing the road it is easy to see how the symptom could arise. The child is taught to be particularly careful when crossing roads and this is emphasized by the need to be accompanied across the road early in life. So in the hierarchy of dangers crossing roads is higher than many others and is recognized as such by young children.

Touching a lamp-post before crossing can give an irrational sense of security; the child feels that in some magical way he is protected from danger when he crosses. Up to this point, a simple behavioural explanation is enough for what we have described. The touching of the lamp-post is the important behaviour. If there is no lamp-post to touch the child is likely to become agitated and anxious, and may have to make a detour to cross the road at another point, so again behaviour is altered. However, the prime mover in this sequence is the superstitious thought, not the behaviour, and until the superstitious thought is altered there is a danger that the behaviour, however it is changed by treatment, will return. What we need to do is to show the child that there is no rational need to touch a lamp-post before crossing the road, that there are other ways of checking whether a road is safe to cross, so that one (slightly) maladaptive behaviour is replaced by an adaptive one.

This problem is not yet severe enough to be a psychiatric disorder but it can easily become one. The option of touching the lamp-post is an attractive and simple one that seems to work, but in the absence of a lamp-post it is clearly inefficient and in an extreme case (a lamp-post-free road) it could prevent crossing the road altogether. Rather than introduce a set of behavioural techniques to extinguish the conditioned behaviour, it is better to introduce a new process, risk management in road crossing, that will ensure safety when crossing (Figure 4.1). This involves a set of appraisal cognitions that can be easily taught (the Highway Code is an example) that properly weigh up the pros and cons of crossing the road and which are much more reliable than touching lamp-posts.

MINDFULNESS CBT

Mindfulness overlaps considerably with mentalization described in the psychodynamic chapter. But the emphasis on thinking and correcting dysfunctional thoughts that is central to cognitive therapy is altered slightly with mindfulness. The notion of mindfulness comes from Buddhist philosophy and is basically concerned with acceptance. Thus it may be possible to have a myriad of unpleasant feelings, thoughts and images that the sufferer wants to have removed. 'You tell me that cognitive behaviour therapy helps to get rid of unpleasant and dysfunctional thoughts; now tell me how I am going to do it?', seems a perfectly reasonable question to ask. But in mindfulness CBT the sufferer is asked to accept these without engaging with them or using what are called distraction techniques to avoid or escape from them. In mindfulness CBT the patient learns to accept these unwelcome thoughts and feelings without paying great attention to them, and by reducing their significance in the person's mind, it is possible for thinking to pass on to other areas which are much less painful and unpleasant. There is now abundant evidence that mindfulness CBT is extremely helpful in a range of mental disorders, particularly depression (Ma and Teasdale, 2004; Kuyken et al., 2008), and this has been said to lead to what has been called the 'third wave' of psychological treatments.

FURTHER EXAMPLES OF THE COGNITIVE BEHAVIOURAL MODEL IN PRACTICE

The example illustrated in Figure 4.1 is not one that is common in clinical practice as lamp-post touchers do not clog child psychiatric clinics yearning for treatment. However, when we examine more common clinical scenarios we find very similar ways of managing more serious problems. Sometimes the behavioural element will predominate, sometimes the cognitive one, but they always interleave and reinforce the other. Let us look at some typical cases and how they are viewed using the cognitive-behavioural model. The format remains the same as with the other models, with the therapist's interpretation in italics.

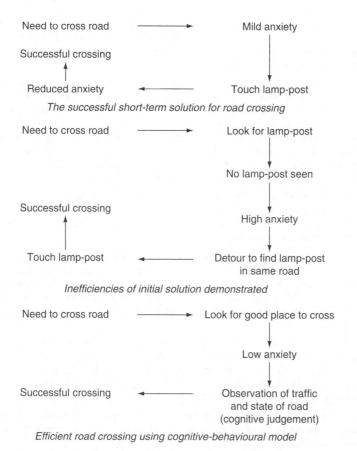

Need to cross road ⟶ Mild anxiety

Successful crossing ⟵ Reduced anxiety ⟵ Touch lamp-post

The successful short-term solution for road crossing

Need to cross road ⟶ Look for lamp-post

No lamp-post seen

High anxiety

Successful crossing ⟵ Touch lamp-post ⟵ Detour to find lamp-post in same road

Inefficiencies of initial solution demonstrated

Need to cross road ⟶ Look for good place to cross

Low anxiety

Successful crossing ⟵ Observation of traffic and state of road (cognitive judgement)

Efficient road crossing using cognitive-behavioural model

Figure 4.1: Simple example of cognitive-behavioural model of road crossing triumphing over lamp-post touching.

THE CASE OF THE ANXIOUS HOUSEWIFE

CASE HISTORY

Presenting problem

A married woman of 23 gives a history of being nervous and frightened about going out of doors since she married her 36-year-old husband four months ago. Symptoms first started after return from honeymoon. She and her husband moved into their new house in a town 40 miles away from her old home where she had lived with her family. She is now afraid to go out of the house alone and feels uneasy travelling with other people apart from her husband.

Interpretation: She has agoraphobic symptoms but these disappear when her husband is with her. He makes her feel secure and allays her anxiety. Looking for her husband when anxious and avoiding going out are two of the 'safety-seeking behaviours' (Salkovskis et al., 1999). This behaviour includes avoidance of a feared situation, escaping from a situation when it is perceived as threatening, and preventing further catastrophe when already in a 'dangerous' situation.

She also sometimes feels frightened when left in the house on her own. Over the past six months she has become progressively more dependent on her husband, a self-employed builder and decorator. He has been very tolerant of her handicap and takes his wife to work with him to reduce her anxiety and accompanies her whenever she goes out shopping. She has tried going out alone on many occasions but each time has acute attacks of panic which prevent her completing her journey and make her feel she is going to pass out. She now refuses to travel by bus or shop in supermarkets alone.

Interpretation: She has developed a conditioned avoidance response. She expects to feel frightened whenever she goes out to shops and therefore avoids it. Each time she avoids going out she reinforces the idea that there is some danger in leaving home alone and therefore the phobia is strengthened.

Her husband is prepared to accompany her whenever necessary and, although he is willing to do this, she feels guilty about having to ask him and is sure he is irritated by her need to do so. She no longer feels as close to her husband as she did before. Matters have not been helped by her reduced sexual interest and at times she has been unable to complete sexual intercourse because of frigidity.

Interpretation: This is a secondary phenomenon (although the psychoanalyst would interpret it as primary since agoraphobia is often thought to be a symbolic fear of sexual intimacy). Her phobias have made her more anxious and insecure. She now feels tense most of the time and always panics when she thinks of going out of the house. Continued reinforcement of the phobia has increased its severity.

Already the therapist has identified an important group of maladaptive symptoms and behaviours that are being magnified by the patient unknowingly.

Family and personal history

Her mother, now aged 49, has always been anxious and has had fears of travelling by train for many years.

Interpretation: Her daughter would almost certainly have been aware of this as a child and imitated her mother to some extent (modelling) in regarding such fears as reasonable and appropriate. She is the younger of two sisters. Her elder sister, four years older, has been married for eight years but is having difficulties in her relationship with her husband and there is talk of separation.

Her father is a regular army commissioned officer who moved frequently during her childhood. This interrupted the patient's schooling and at times she had short episodes of refusing to go to school following transfer to a different part of the country.

Interpretation: These were the first signs of her adult phobic symptoms, which often appear about the age of 11 (Tyrer and Tyrer, 1974). One of these episodes lasted for two weeks, during which she had severe headaches and had episodes of vomiting and the school attendance officer had to be called in.

According to her school reports she always underachieved at school and appeared to be uncomfortable there. She had few friends, passed no examinations and left aged 15.

Previous personality

Has always been anxious and shy and found it difficult to make friends. The friends she has made have been very close and she has tended to rely on them a great deal. Prefers an ordered life and her hobbies include knitting and crocheting, crossword puzzles and watching television. Smokes 15 cigarettes a day.

Interpretation: This type of anxious fearful personality is prone to maladaptive conditioning. Once patterns of behaviour are established they are difficult to break and she has probably had anxious cognitions over a long period.

Mental state

Appearance and behaviour: She presented as a carefully made-up young woman who was anxious during interview, frequently smoothed back her hair and flicked imaginary pieces of fluff off her clothes. Restless, frequently adjusted her position throughout interview as though sitting on blunt drawing pins. Speech: Talked rapidly in a soft voice although became less nervous during interview. Inhibited about her sexual difficulties and preferred talking at length about her phobic symptoms, which she insisted lay behind all her difficulties.

Interpretation: This is a correct interpretation. Once her phobic symptoms are treated she will feel more secure and her sexual difficulties will resolve. The dynamic therapist would continue to probe with further questions and would be determined to find a link with her symptoms, whether or not such a link was justified.

The formal diagnosis of the condition is clearly agoraphobia, together with panic attacks in the feared situations. Its treatment will consist of a combination of approaches that change cognition and behaviour. The cognitive component shows that in our agoraphobic patient there is a very low threshold to the appraisal of threat or danger. She genuinely believes that, when she is having her panic attack in the street, she is threatened with either physical or social harm. It does not matter that to others this fear is unjustified. It does not require a *real* threat to be present for the *experience* of anxiety to be intense and debilitating. In cognitive therapy the understanding of this phenomenon is the first step in reminding the patient that the false reassurance of there is nothing to worry about' is of no value when you are having a panic attack and interpret the symptoms as those of imminent collapse. Although our patient has made a cognitive error in believing she is about to collapse when she is having a panic attack her experience may be very similar to that of a person who is actually about to lose consciousness.

The behavioural element of treatment will consist of extinguishing the conditioned avoidance response by gradual exposure to the feared situations along the lines discussed earlier. Some of this treatment may require little tasks or behavioural experiments (Salkovskis and Hackmann, 1997) to test progress. Thus, for example, after initial progress in overcoming her panics by breaking the loop that connects feelings of panic with an impending heart attack, our agoraphobic patient is asked to keep a diary of her anxious feelings to develop a 'personal fingerprint' of her anxiety. She is convinced that this will show no consistent pattern, but the results show that she is habitually less anxious in the late afternoon in the hour before her husband returns home from work. The reasons for this can only be guessed at, but in practice the journey alone to the supermarket at 4 p.m. is a useful experiment to test out the possibility that this is a favourable time of day for exposure to phobic stimuli.

In psychodynamic therapy a great deal is attached to transference and countertransference in treatment. The relative unimportance of this in the cognitive-behavioural model is illustrated by the success of this approach when given interactively through a computer terminal (Proudfoot *et al.*, 2003). As treatment programs improve this may be the favoured way of delivering such therapy.

THE CASE OF THE HYPOCHONDRIACAL DEPRESSIVE

Our anxious housewife had a clear behavioural problem, agoraphobia, that is recognized to be appropriate for the cognitive-behavioural model. Now let us look at a more complicated problem in which depression and hypochondriasis (health anxiety) are prominent features.

CASE HISTORY

Presenting Problem

A 29-year-old woman, referred to the psychiatrist by her general practitioner with recurrent anxiety and depressive symptoms complicated by concerns about her health. Part of his letter read: 'she often calls me out in the evening or presents to the casualty department in the middle of the night, convinced she is having a heart attack, and although I have reassured her that all the tests are normal and she has no evidence of any heart disease she does not believe me. I am frustrated with her and she is frustrated with me. She has become more depressed recently and says that she cannot go on feeling like this. I am particularly concerned now because she has threatened suicide if there is no hope of an end to her troubles.'

Interpretation: She misinterprets the attacks as heart disease but as they continue in the absence of any explanation of her symptoms she has her opinions reinforced. It is not surprising that she has become depressed.

History of condition

Well until nine months previously. Had an acute attack of palpitations and sweating while resting at home after a busy day. During this attack was convinced she would pass out and thought that she might be having a heart attack. Called out her doctor, who came to see her within half-an-hour, examined her and could find nothing wrong. By this time she had recovered from her attack and was not surprised that the doctor found nothing of significance, and so she responded to his reassurance. Four days later she had another attack while sitting at a word processor at her work at a bank where she was a senior secretary. She had the same palpitations and sweating and when, after about five minutes, she started feeling that she was going to collapse she was again convinced that her doctor must have been wrong and she was having a heart attack. Her work colleagues saw her in this state and agreed that there must be something seriously wrong. An occupational health nurse saw her immediately and rushed her to a local casualty department. She was examined fully by several doctors in the department and had a range of further tests, including electrocardiograms. A heart murmur was noted and she was advised to come back for further tests at a cardiology clinic.

Interpretation: Her suspicion that she might have a heart condition has been reinforced by her work colleagues and an occupational health nurse, so she is now convinced her original thinking was correct.

Further progress

The tests confirmed no significant cardiac pathology and she was again reassured. Now was convinced that the doctors must be wrong because she was having attacks four times a week. Could never predict an attack and was angry when her general practitioner suggested they might be related to stress. She described clearly that they occurred without warning in many situations, often when she was sitting relaxed in a chair. Recently had also developed pain in the lower ribs and this had confirmed her view that she had a heart condition.

Interpretation: She does not have any explanation for her symptoms and a quoted link with 'stress' has no explanatory meaning behind it, so she finds the pain in her ribs a more plausible association, reinforcing her belief that she has heart disease.

Initial treatment

The general practitioner suggested referring her to his practice nurse for counselling, but this was rejected angrily by the patient who insisted that her continued problem was not a psychological one. However, her attacks continued; she became demoralized and depressed. Could see no future, and at times did not mind if she died in one of her attacks as at least this would 'solve the problem'. Saw no point in living while her attacks continued and became preoccupied by guilt about consulting her general practitioner so frequently. When she said to him that she was becoming a burden on his practice and might it not be better if she were dead he became alarmed and persuaded her to be referred to the psychiatrist.

Interpretation: She is now becoming significantly depressed and again is demonstrating misinterpretation of her symptoms that is predictable with the cognitive-behavioural model. It is now time to use the model positively to change her thinking and behaviour.

Treatment using the cognitive model

To illustrate the working of the model in actual practice it is useful to record verbatim the interaction between the cognitive therapist and the patient. She came into the clinic room looking miserable and glum and it was clear she was obviously depressed.

PATIENT: 'I'm sorry to bother you but my doctor insisted I came. But you'll be like all the others; you won't find anything wrong with me and say there's nothing the matter. Not that I'm worth helping anyway.'

THERAPIST: 'If you aren't worth helping why do you think your doctor referred you to the clinic?'

PATIENT: 'He just wanted to get me off his hands. My friends are the same. They don't want to talk to me any more; I'm such a pain. They just want me to disappear from their lives.'

THERAPIST: 'What makes you think that?'

PATIENT: 'Because they stay out of my way. They avoid talking to me unless they have to. I think they realize I've got a fatal illness and feel embarrassed when they're with me.'

THERAPIST: 'What makes you feel you have a fatal illness?'

PATIENT: 'I get these attacks of palpitations and sweating and know it's a heart attack but noone believes me.'

THERAPIST: 'I can understand your feelings. But could I just check with you if there are any other possible causes of palpitations and sweating. If you had a twin sister who came to you and said she had palpitations and sweating, what could be the possible causes apart from a heart attack?'

PATIENT: 'Well, I do have a sister and she gets sweating attacks and has palpitations occasionally, but she has diabetes.'

THERAPIST: 'All right, I agree, diabetes. Any other possibilities?'

PATIENT: 'I suppose my son gets like this when he watches his favourite team, Leicester City, on the television. He gets so worked up when they let in a goal; you'd think it was the end of the world.'

THERAPIST: 'So the stress of watching the game would bring on the symptoms?'

PATIENT: 'Yes. My uncle Ron used to get the palpitations too. He worked down the mines and had that lung disease, pneumoconi something. And my sister also gets all sweaty whenever she has those funny little fish in food – what are they called – anchovies – because she's got an allergy to them.'

THERAPIST: 'Well we have quite a few possibilities now. Now could I just have your help in an exercise. If you were to put yourself in my position and 100 patients were to come to see me in the next few days with palpitations and sweating, according to your experience, some might have diabetes, some might be having a heart attack, some may be in stressful situations and some might be having allergic reactions.'

PATIENT: 'Yes, but of course I'm not an expert.'

THERAPIST: 'Well could you help me guess at the likely number in each group, starting with the most common?' (As the patient responds the therapist draws a diagram that shows the proportions roughly – see Figure 4.2).

THERAPIST: 'So here we have the results; they are very encouraging for me. Less than one in ten people with palpitations and sweating are likely to be suffering from a heart attack, so I will have much less to do than I might have thought when they come in.'

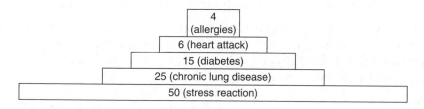

Figure 4.2:   The patient's view of the likely causes of palpitations and sweating in 100 consecutively referred patients to a clinic.

The therapist ends the session with a formulation of the problem that can be copied and taken home by the patient to reinforce the progress made in this first interview. One of the best ways of doing this is to take the patient to a recent episode when she was very fearful about her health. Once this is identified, the day, exact time, situation and activity need to be noted. So the conversation might go along these lines:

PATIENT: 'I had just got back from work, arriving back at an empty house. I was annoyed that the new manager did not seem to recognize the amount of effort I had put into some recent work. I was making a cup of tea and I noticed I was getting sweaty. I began to feel scared, and thought, "oh no, not again". I checked my pulse; it was faster than usual, and I was expecting palpitations. I walked across the kitchen and looked in the mirror – I noticed I looked pale, and got even more anxious and felt I was going to have a heart attack.'

THERAPIST: 'What was going through your mind at that time? What would it mean to have a heart attack?'

PATIENT: 'I'd die a horrible death – just like that.'

THERAPIST: 'And did you have images that came into your mind at that time?'

PATIENT: 'Yes, my funeral.'

THERAPIST: 'And what do you see?'

PATIENT: 'The coffin being lowered into the ground and hardly anyone being there.'

THERAPIST: 'Why would there be few people there?'

PATIENT: 'Because I haven't had a chance to find the right man – I know my ex wouldn't be there.'

THERAPIST: 'And what would dying mean for you?'

PATIENT: 'I've never lived, or had children, or seen them growing up.'

THERAPIST: 'So when you get these feelings that you are going to have a heart attack, it's not just the fear of the attack that is troubling you here; it's a feeling you haven't fulfilled many of the things you wanted to do in life. We have to take this into account as well.'

The subsequent management might include the patient completing diaries of the times she has these episodes and the relevant thoughts that may be in both the foreground and the background at that time.

If you would like to read more about this approach, it is available in book form (Tyrer, 2013).

FUNDAMENTAL DIFFERENCES BETWEEN THE COGNITIVE-BEHAVIOURAL MODEL AND OTHER MODELS

To see the important differences between the cognitive-behavioural model and others it is just necessary to examine this conversation again closely. You will notice that the interaction between patient and therapist has changed during the course of the interview. The patient begins by expecting a combination of pointless questions that she does not believe are the ones the therapist wants to ask, and (what she perceives as) empty reassurance that there is nothing significantly wrong with her. By the end of the interview she has helped to persuade the therapist (but possibly not yet herself) that most people with palpitations and sweating are not likely to be suffering from a heart attack.

This type of interchange is very common when the cognitive-behavioural model is used in treatment. It is a good example of an empirically grounded clinical intervention (Salkovskis, 2002) that gently explores the beliefs of the patient (and the therapist) and gradually brings them towards a common pathway. In subsequent parts of treatment it will probably be necessary to explore the symptoms of depression that have begun to have an influence on the problem and the same approach will be used.

The assumption that nobody cares about her (despite some evidence to the contrary) is a depressive cognition that needs to be challenged. For the adherents of the disease model, these depressive thoughts are a direct consequence of the biochemical disturbances lying behind depressive illness. For the cognitive therapist, however, these thoughts are seen to lead clearly to increasing levels of depression, or, more commonly, its perpetuation and development. Rather than contradicting the patient (the approach that has conspicuously failed from the beginning of her illness), the therapist will explore what has actually been happening and thereby directly challenge the patient's assumption that she is disliked and ignored. In further discussions the patient repeated the same negative line of thinking when describing her doctor's attitude. She had interpreted his comments that there was nothing seriously wrong with her physical health as a direct contradiction of her own feelings. 'He kept saying there was nothing wrong,' she said, 'but I knew the way I felt. I was having these attacks when I felt awful and never had them before, so obviously something was wrong.' She had gone further in her depressive thinking by interpreting the doctor's reassurance about her physical health as a wish to dismiss her from the surgery as she was becoming a nuisance. First she blamed the doctor for what she construed as misdiagnosis, but later she blamed herself. (One of the reasons for this is that as she became more depressed her panic attacks disappeared. She therefore thought that perhaps her symptoms during these attacks might have been less real than she at first thought and that perhaps she was to blame for bothering the doctor). In dealing with the depressive symptoms the therapist may also bring in behaviour therapy in some form. Since the time of Charles Darwin, who suffered from serious depression, it has been recognized that positive behavioural activity helps the symptoms and this has now been formalized as behavioural activation treatment, and shown to be effective (Ekers *et al.*, 2011).

Our case histories illustrate that in the cognitive-behavioural model the therapist is genuinely interested in symptoms and behaviour because they are the fundamentals in therapy. There is a general feeling that people who talk about their personal symptoms of illness are the ultimate bores; nobody listening wants to hear about them and only stay listening because in pleasurable anticipation they are waiting for the chance to start on their own round of complaints. Well, and you may need reminding about this, in the cognitive-behavioural arena the listeners do want to hear. They want to know every single symptom and, more particularly, the beliefs and thoughts associated with them, as these will help understanding and probably play a role in treatment at some time.

In the other models symptoms and behaviour are also-rans in the process of assessment and care. In the disease model they are merely signposts to a disease label; in the psychodynamic model they are symbolic clues (so the demonstration of agoraphobic symptoms and frigidity are both recognized by dream analysts as symbolic of aversion to sexual intercourse), and in the social model we return to symptoms and behaviour as labels of an alleged medical condition which really has a social cause. The cognitive-behavioural model is a very versatile one and, in addition to the conditions we have already described, it has been applied successfully to eating disorders (Freeman *et al.*, 1988), personality disorder (Beck, 1991; Davidson and Tyrer, 1996; Davidson *et al.*, 2010), alcohol and drug abuse, disorders of sleep and other problems of physiological functions, and marital disorders (Schmaling *et al.*, 1989). The approach will be evident from the general principles of the model. Thus the central preoccupation of the anorexic girl that her body is obscenely fat, the patient with the personality disorder whose close relationships keep on breaking down but in every case it is always someone else's fault, the alcoholic who thinks that whenever he feels depressed alcohol will cheer him up, and the insomniac who feels that he never sleeps a wink and will die from perpetual wakefulness, all have similar dysfunctional thoughts. The adaptive, appropriate, rational thoughts are not easy to substitute for the irrational ones, but it can be done by the collaborative, empirical approach of cognitive therapy.

A useful analogy is to think of a team of horses pulling a coach. Normally the coachman is in control and the horses stay still, trot or gallop at the coachman's command. But in these disorders the horses are out of control; the coachman can do nothing except warn the passengers to take evading action and hope that the horses will come to their senses before they or the people on the coach suffer serious injury. The cognitive therapist is represented by the rider who gallops alongside the horses, calms them down and helps them to find an alternative less frantic form of motion that is more comfortable to them and the people about them, so that eventually they come under the coachman's (adaptive) control again.

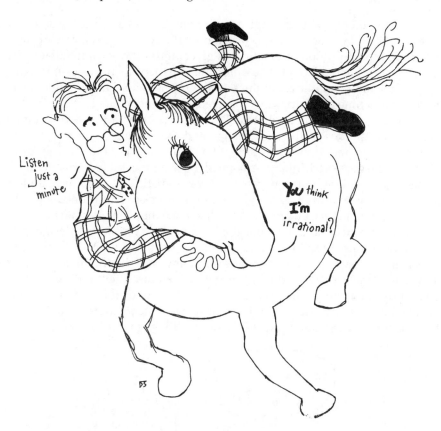

OTHER APPLICATIONS OF THE COGNITIVE-BEHAVIOURAL MODEL

Our phobic patient was treated by counter-conditioning but classical and operant conditioning are also used in treatment. Classical conditioning is best represented in the form of aversion therapy. For example, the continual excessive drinking of the alcoholic is maladaptive because it leads to further drinking (through dependence) (Ghodse and Maxwell, 1990) and increased problems in living. Unfortunately the harm caused by alcohol abuse is delayed whilst its immediate effect is often pleasurable. It follows from the laws of conditioning that drinking behaviour therefore tends to be reinforced. The maladaptive response is 'alcohol is good for you', and in the short term it seems to solve many of life's problems. In aversion therapy a highly unpleasant negative stimulus-response pattern is placed as close as possible to the reinforcing maladaptive one in the expectation that the two will link together. If this happens the drinking of alcohol becomes associated with nasty feelings that overcome the former pleasurable ones.

In aversion therapy for alcohol abuse, vomiting is the most commonly induced negative response. An injection or drink of a drug which causes vomiting (apomorphine or emetine) is given and followed immediately by the consumption of alcohol. The unfortunate patient then passes through a cycle of retching, vomiting, giddiness and wretchedness. To add authenticity to the proceedings the drinking is staged in a congenial setting, with soft lights, music and general bonhomie. But as soon as the nausea and vomiting begins the attitudes of the staff change and the sufferer is berated for the squalor and degradation he has brought on himself, and which will continue as long as he goes on drinking. An outsider seeing this little drama might be excused for thinking that the treatment was sadistic and inhumane and its sole object was to humiliate the victim of the exercise. This immediate reaction is understandable, but when it is realized that the alcoholic is an informed partner to the treatment and that the behaviour of the staff is designed to maximize negative reinforcement, ultimately for the patient's benefit, such criticism evaporates. The treatment can, in any case, be modified to avoid vomiting while still producing negative reinforcement (Blake, 1965). Dialectical behaviour therapy, a highly structured form of cognitive-behavioural therapy with additional components, has also been modified to treat alcohol and substance misuse disorders (Linehan *et al.*, 2002).

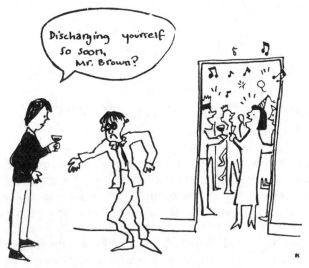

'To add authenticity to the proceedings...'

The cognitive-behavioural model is also widely used with clinical problems in children and those with intellectual disability. A behaviour such as feeding oneself without help is often a major hurdle for the handicapped child. In the past, inability to carry out self-feeding (and similar behaviour which the intellectually normal child does not think twice about) was accepted as part and parcel of mental handicap. Now we realize that the potential to achieve greater independence is present in many of these children. Combinations of empirically grounded interventions and simple reinforcement can be used to maximize abilities that might otherwise lie dormant. This is not as easy as it sounds, for it is difficult not to give the incompetent child more attention than the successful one, and attention is a powerful reinforcer. In other types of abnormal behaviour, particularly those which are destructive and disruptive, stronger negative reinforcement may be used.

A therapist well-trained in learning theory and cognitive therapy is able to design a programme for treating every sort of abnormal behaviour. The first part of assessment is to find out if there are any precipitants of the behaviour and whether it is predictable (a behavioural or functional analysis). Responses that lessen or increase the behaviour (positive and negative reinforcers) are then studied, and a good behavioural modification programme should have an approximately even number of these. The idea that behaviourists have a penchant to punish is a myth; they much prefer to reward. A cognitive-behavioural programme is constructed and all personnel involved with the client, be they parents, children, nurses or doctors, are seen and agreement reached collaboratively on how it should be run. This is important, because if there is inconsistency between the different personnel involved with treatment its effectiveness will be greatly reduced.

CRITICISMS OF THE COGNITIVE-BEHAVIOURAL MODEL AND THEIR REBUTTAL

The critics of the cognitive-behavioural model feel the claims for its application and value have been overstated. They view it as a rather fancy way of telling the patient to 'think a bit more about what you're doing' (cognitive element) and 'pull yourself together' (behavioural element), coated with layers of jargon. The assertion that the symptoms and behaviour are the essentials of mental illness is one that particularly irritates the advocate of the psychodynamic model. What is shown to the dynamic psychotherapist as behaviour is only the end product of a complicated series of processes involving the conscious and unconscious mind. To claim that abnormal behaviour is synonymous with illness ignores all these factors. A man who intends to commit suicide, drives to a high cliff and then jumps to his death only shows abnormal behaviour in the last seconds of his life, but the mental processes that led to his suicide preceded the behaviour by many weeks or months. If the suicide leap was prevented by a temporary form of positive reinforcement, or delayed by a cognitive arrow targeted at hopeless-ness, it would only be repeated later in another form if the underlying conflict were not resolved. Behaviourism linked to appropriate cognitions is just not enough to explain the creative genius of Beethoven, Shakespeare, Leonardo da Vinci and Michelangelo. It is laughable to pretend that their work was just the end-product of conditioned and unconditioned reflexes, of well-posi-tioned positive and negative reinforcement, as otherwise we could all achieve the same powers.

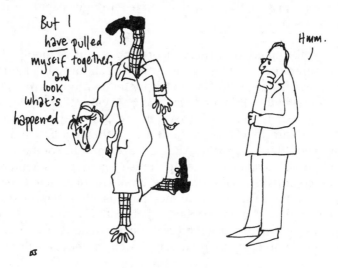

'… pull yourself together…'

The cognitive-behavioural therapist acknowledges these attacks, but answers that the cognitive-behavioural model is not a prescription for the human con-dition, but is concerned simply with maladaptive thinking and functioning. Adaptive functioning is gloriously varied; maladaptive functioning tends to be stereotyped. There is an easy reply to the Shavian criticism that all the principles of behaviour therapy are self-evident and require no special knowledge; there are many common-sense ways of dealing with problems that are quite inappropriate and lead to maladaptive learning. The mother who goes and cuddles her child every time she shows the slightest distress is very likely to set up an attention-seeking pattern of response. The child who is rewarded by a cuddle whenever she is upset may either use such behaviour as a manipulative gesture or may become excessively dependent and clinging.

The man who burgles a house and is caught in the act does not get punished immediately. He usually appears in court and is released on bail. Many weeks later he goes on trial and may go to prison. The negative reinforcement of imprisonment is far removed in time from the crime and we know from learning theory that any unconditioned response that develops will be a weak one. But what happens if the burglar is not caught? He gets positive reinforcement immediately when he escapes with his loot. So it is hardly surprising that petty thieving becomes a career, and we breed recidivists, apparently incorrigible rogues who are 'incapable of learning right from wrong.' Of course they are quite capable of learning correctly but we need to alter the associations between reward and punishment for it to be effective.

As the cognitive-behavioural model develops, more complex techniques are introduced which are far removed from simple Pavlovian conditioning or the correction and adjustment of dysfunctional thoughts. Modelling, of which mention has already been made, involves showing the ideal form of behaviour to a client (e.g. showing a film of a calm patient receiving dental treatment) and another, shaping, involves reinforcing successively closer approximations to the required response. More complex belief systems, or schemas (Young, 1994), are more difficult to alter than isolated thoughts and require different modifications of the cognitive-behavioural model. However much we try to forget it, our complex and apparently original behaviour is composed of many smaller units of behaviour which obey certain established laws. This is no different from saying that deep down we all have the same basic structural unit, the double helix of the DNA molecule. Why no-one takes exception to this, yet waxes eloquently about the over-simplification of cognitive-behavioural theory, is beyond rational comprehension.

The cognitive-behavioural model is also at odds with the disease model on many issues. Often it finds (e.g. in health anxiety) that the sick role is inappropriate for many psychological disorders, and may contribute to handicap. Worse still, it may create new illness (i.e. is iatrogenic). By adopting a passive role the patient is rewarded by the medical model. Like a lump of clay on the potter's wheel he is moulded into a shape chosen by the doctor. This shape may be right or quite wrong, but it is more likely to be the latter, as the doctor is limited by his organic orientation and through his blinkered eyes can only recognize disease. Our clay patient is returned to society in his new mould only to return sharply when he realizes he still does not fit. So a cycle of admission and relapses follows (about half of all psychiatric in-patients are readmitted to hospital) until either the doctor or patient retires through exhaustion.

If doctors were a profession provoking abuse and disdain the attention would not be rewarding, but as things stand at present all such attention positively reinforces the sick role. So the independent person becomes a passive patient. At subsequent consultation and relapses his power to shape his own destiny is gradually whittled away until he no longer thinks or acts independently; this reaches its final form in the stereotyped institutional behaviour of the chronic hospitalized patient, now a relatively rare occurrence. This state has been reproduced in animals when they are placed in situations where others decide what happens to them. It is an apathetic, sad condition now often called learned helplessness. Doctors who follow the disease model unwittingly encourage helplessness and may thereby promote new 'illness.'

The hierarchy of medicine is alien to the behavioural therapist. There is no need for an authoritarian approach in the cognitive-behavioural model. The person with the necessary skills is the one who organizes the treatment. Others in a team may be involved in carrying out the programme (and specially trained nurses are often essential) but a two-way contract between treaters and treated cannot develop in a hierarchical atmosphere. It is no good telling patients that a treatment is to be given because the expert has decided that this is the best available. No good treatment will be effective unless the reasons for choosing it are explained and cooperation obtained. So it is in everyone's interests to have an informal relationship between the parties concerned and to avoid the pronouncements of authority. Moreover, the goals and methods, and indeed the rationale, of the cognitive-behavioural model can be readily discussed in plain language by therapist and patient.

The adherent to the cognitive-behavioural model is also able to dismiss another bogey that is frequently resurrected when the model's therapy is being criticized, that of *symptom substitution*. This concept has developed from psychodynamic theory, particularly from the 'hydraulic' concepts of Freud. Symptoms, according to Freud, are the unhealthy expression of libidinous forces. These forces would be expressed differently if the ego and superego allowed them to come out into the open. Because they are repressed and denied they resurface in an alien form, psychiatric symptoms, which are acceptable to the ego because they completely disguise the real problem. It therefore follows that if these symptoms are merely regarded as the illness in its entirety, and treatment focused only on removing them, the problem is going to resurface in another form. Like the hydra of Greek mythology, if one head is chopped off two new ones will grow in its place. So new symptoms will be substituted for old ones and until the therapist explores more deeply no real progress will be made.

The behaviourist notes this theoretical criticism. Instead of responding in kind with an equally plausible defence of symptomatic treatment he turns to the empirical evidence. When follow-up studies of behaviour therapy are examined there is no evidence that symptom substitution occurs to any appreciable extent (Emmelkamp and Kuipers, 1979). If there is a return of symptoms it is almost always of the same nature as the original symptoms. Symptom substitution is largely a myth and should not be a reason for not treating symptoms directly.

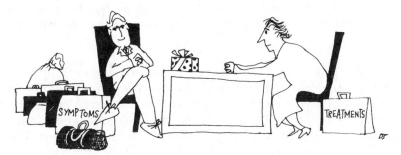

'So new symptoms will be substituted for old ones...'

The advocates of the social model are also unhappy about the spread of the cognitive-behavioural model, but for different reasons. The concept of conditioning and cognitive control worries them because, although they may at first be used to remove unpleasant symptoms, they can easily be manipulated to induce conformity. For example, homosexuality was formerly considered a criminal offence (as well as a disease in the official classification of disease) but in our more enlightened times is accepted as part of normal variation. Behaviour therapy in the past certainly has not helped the cause of enlightenment, as it was used to argue the case that homosexuality is a form of abnormal behaviour that needs to be extinguished. In its simplest form the client is negatively reinforced (e.g. by receiving an electric shock) whenever he shows a sexual response (e.g. engorgement of the penis recorded by a blood flow measurement called penile plethysmography) to a nude photograph of a member of his own sex and positively reinforced by similar responses to the opposite sex. The homosexual response is therefore treated as deviant and unhealthy. The techniques of brainwashing have been developed along the same lines and people can be forced to believe things and behave in ways that are entirely alien to them. However, this sort of argument follows from the effectiveness of behaviour therapy, not its supposed moral or political position. If someone wished to change his sexual orientation, or any other preference, the cognitive-behavioural model offers an effective, voluntary means of doing so, but it should never be forced on anyone.

The cognitive-behaviourist is aware of the powers that his treatment possesses but can claim with justification that, although all successful therapies can be abused, this is not a reason for abandoning them. He can also emphasize that in the therapeutic use of behaviour therapy the patient should be motivated to come for treatment and not be dragooned by an external agency.

This is not just pious talk, because those who come for behaviour therapy against their will, be they homosexual, phobic or obsessional, will show little or no response. It is only in a society entirely ruled by Orwellian conformity that brainwashing would be commonplace and it is up to us as political beings to ensure that such a society never develops. But it would be quite wrong to deprive psychology of an effective treatment because of this potential danger.

The cognitive-behavioural model brings psychiatric disorders out from the murky caves of dynamic theory and examines them in the light of day. It records and treats what it observes, and scorns conjecture. Most psychiatric disorder is grist to its mill because it consists of abnormal behaviour and symptoms rather than disease. It has a firm, scientific base in experimental psychology and this enables it to plan and predict the effects of treatment instead of relying on empiricism alone. Although it is a relatively recent newcomer to psychiatry, its supporters are confident it will become the major impetus for progress in the future. Tomorrow's students of psychiatry will need to know much more of cognitive dysfunction and learning theory and less of the minutiae of disease if they are to become effective practitioners; and despite its adaptability and sophistication its principles are logical and straightforward.

PUTTING THE PATIENT IN CONTROL

The cognitive-behavioural model is the most recent of the models described in this book and it is therefore not surprising that it is the one that is most receptive to patients. The spirit of collaboration that permeates the model allows both therapist and patient to set off on a journey together in exploring symptoms that are at first mysterious but which later are understood and conquered. Cognitive-behavioural therapy, although introduced by a psychiatrist, Tim Beck, is now practised much more by psychologists and other professionals such as nurses than by doctors. I personally think that one of the problems that doctors have in practising cognitive-behavioural therapy is that they are used to telling patients what is wrong with them. This didactic approach is not part of the cognitive model. In the best form of treatment the patient finds out what is wrong with them through the treatment, not through being told, but by working it out for themselves. This process is sometimes called 'guided discovery.'

This approach can often be a revelation to people who have suffered for years without getting over to any person they have consulted over this time what it is like to have their symptoms. For example, we have recently seen someone who has had an obsessive-compulsive disorder for over twenty years.

This condition has a tendency to be persistent and is characterized by excessive doubt and the need to check things and carry out actions (rituals) or thoughts (ruminations) repeatedly, even though these activities are recognized to be unnecessary and to some extent are resisted. However, if the rituals and ruminations are not carried out the sufferer becomes intolerably anxious as he or she feels that some disaster will occur for which their personal responsibility will be total.

The symptoms in this particular case included doubts about contamination (hands had to be kept close to the body when walking past people in case accidental contact could be interpreted as molestation), injury to others (e.g. when overtaking a cyclist by car there was doubt whether a collision might have occurred, so the driver had to stop the car and wait for the cyclist to catch up and prove to the driver they were still alive) and the need to examine blemishes on his face for periods of up to six hours at a time to make sure they were not expanding and becoming cancerous.

These symptoms are now being systematically explored, tested and treated by the cognitive-behavioural model. At this stage it is impossible to say how long this will take and what will be the outcome, not least as resistant obsessional disorder is very difficult to treat. Even at this stage, however, what has happened to the patient is little short of a fundamental revelation. For the first time he has been able to talk freely about his symptoms in an understanding setting and to appreciate that they are not fixed obstacles around which he has to negotiate but problems that have the potential to be removed. He has also appreciated that he is not unique: everybody has intrusive thoughts and it is the response to these that determines whether they become part of a mental disorder or accepted as part of the humdrum nature of existence.

He now has some framework on which to operate in dealing with his symptoms. And because he is testing each new approach himself, admittedly with external help (often called guided discovery), he feels in control and a central player in the treatment process. This is of great help for the future as, if he does get better but, as sometimes happens, he has a relapse and a return of his symptoms they will not be regarded as catastrophic. The same approach can be tried again in different forms and again the patient takes control, often before any professional input is given. In practice this means that serious relapse is less common after treatment with the cognitive-behavioural model than after treatment using other models (e.g. the disease one) when the patient has less responsibility for its successful treatment (Evans *et al.*, 1992).

So our patient, and the many others who have benefited from this model over the years, is like a visitor to a foreign country who has not been able to understand the language of his hosts. When suddenly he begins to appreciate the words and phrases in common use a whole new vista of experience and understanding opens in front of him. Much of what has been uncertain and alien now becomes familiar and homely, strangers kept at bay by a communication barrier now become friends, and fears and doubts are replaced by the warmness of certainty and support. The language of the cognitive-behavioural model is not difficult to learn and it will yield similar dividends.

REFERENCES

Beck, A.T. (1976) *Cognitive Therapy and the Emotional Disorders.* International Universities Press, New York.

Beck, A.T. (1991) *Cognitive Therapy of Personality Disorders.* Guilford Press, New York.

Beck, A.T. (2006) How an anomalous finding led to a new system of psychotherapy. *Nature Medicine*, **12**, 1139–1141.

Beck, A.T., Emery, G. and Greenberg, R. (1985) *Anxiety Disorders and Phobias: a Cognitive Perspective.* Basic Books, New York.

Blackburn, I.M. and Davidson, K.M. (1995) *Cognitive Therapy for Depression and Anxiety.* Blackwell Scientific, Oxford.

Blake, B.G. (1965) The application of behaviour therapy to the treatment of alcoholism. *Behaviour Research and Therapy*, **3**, 75–80.

Davidson, K.M. and Tyrer, P. (1996) Cognitive therapy for antisocial and borderline personality disorder: single case study series. *British Journal of Clinical Psychology*, **35**, 413–429.

Davidson, K.M., Tyrer, P., Norrie, J., Palmer, S.J., and Tyrer, H. (2010). Cognitive therapy v. usual treatment for borderline personality disorder: prospective 6-year follow-up. *British Journal of Psychiatry*, **197**, 456–462.

Ekers, D., Richards, D., McMillan, D., Bland, J.M., and Gilbody, S. (2011). Behavioural activation delivered by the non-specialist: phase II randomised controlled trial. *British Journal of Psychiatry*, **198**, 66–72.

Ellis, A. (1962) *Reason and Emotion in Psychotherapy.* Stuart, New York.

Ellis, A. (1995) Changing rational-emotive therapy (RET) to rational emotive behavior therapy (REBT). *Journal of Rational-Emotive and Cognitive-Behavior Therapy*, **13**, 85–90.

Emmelkamp, P.M.G. and Kuipers, A.C.M. (1979) Agoraphobia: a follow-up study 4 years after treatment. *British Journal of Psychiatry*, **134**, 352–355.

Evans, M.D., Hollon, S.D., *et al.* (1992) Differential relapse following cognitive therapy and pharmacotherapy for depression. *Archives of General Psychiatry*, **49**, 802–808.

Freeman, C.P., Barry, F., *et al.* (1988) Controlled trial of psychotherapy for bulimia nervosa. *British Medical Journal*, **296**, 521–525.

Ghodse, A.H. and Maxwell, D. (1990) *Substance Misuse and Dependence: An Introduction for the Caring Professions.* Macmillan, London.

Kingdon, D. and Turkington, D. (1993) *Cognitive Therapy in Schizophrenia.* Guilford Press, New York.

Kuyken, W., Byford, S., Taylor, R.S., *et al.* (2008). Mindfulness-based cognitive therapy to prevent relapse in recurrent depression. *Journal of Consulting and Clinical Psychology*, **76**, 966–978.

Linehan, M.M., Dimeff, L.A., Reynolds, S.K., *et al.* (2002) Dialectical behavior therapy versus comprehensive validation therapy plus 12-step for the treatment of opioid dependent women meeting criteria for borderline personality disorder. *Drug and Alcohol Dependence*, **67**, 13–26.

Ma, S.H. and Teasdale, J.D. (2004) Mindfulness-based cognitive therapy for depression: replication and exploration of differential relapse prevention effects. *Journal of Consulting and Clinical Psychology*, **72**, 31–40.

Orwell, G. (1949) *1984*. Secker and Warburg, London.

Pavlov, I.P. (1927) *Conditioned Reflexes*. Oxford University Press, London.

Pavlov, I.P. (1941) *Conditioned Reflexes and Psychiatry*. International Publishers, New York.

Perry, A., Tarrier, N., Morriss, R., McCarthy, E. and Limb, K. (1999) Randomised controlled trial of efficacy of teaching patients with bipolar disorder to identify early symptoms of relapse and obtain treatment. *British Medical Journal*, **318**, 149–153.

Proudfoot, J., Goldberg, D., Mann, A., Everitt, B., Marks, I., and Gray, J.A. (2003) Computerized, interactive, multimedia cognitive-behavioural program for anxiety and depression in general practice. *Psychological Medicine*, **33**, 217–227.

Ryle, A. (1997) The structure and development of borderline personality disorder: a proposed model. *British Journal of Psychiatry*, **170**, 82–87.

Salkovskis, P.M. (2002) Empirically grounded clinical interventions: cognitivebehavioural therapy progresses through a multi-dimensional approach to clinical science. *Behavioural and Cognitive Psychotherapy*, **30**, 3–9.

Salkovskis, P.M., and Hackmann, A. (1997) Agoraphobia. In: G.C.L. Davey (ed.), *Phobias: A Handbook of Theory, Research and Treatment*, pp. 27–62. Wiley, Chichester.

Salkovskis, P.M., Clark, D.M., Hackmann, A., Wells, A. and Gelder, M.G. (1999) An experimental investigation of the role of safety-seeking behaviours in the maintenance of panic disorder with agoraphobia. *Behaviour Research and Therapy*, **37**, 559–574.

Schmaling, K.B., Fruzzetti, A.E. and Jacobson, N.S. (1989) Marital problems. In: K. Hawton, P.M. Salkovskis, J. Kirk and D.M. Clark (eds) *Cognitive Behaviour Therapy for Psychiatric Problems*, pp. 339–369. Oxford Medical, Oxford.

Shaw, G.B. (1932) *The Adventures of the Black Girl in Her Search for God*. Constable, London.

Skinner, B.F. (1972) *Beyond Freedom and Dignity*. Jonathan Cape, London.

Tyrer, H. (2013) *Tackling Health Anxiety: a CBT Handbook*. RCPsych Press, London.

Tyrer, P. and Tyrer, S. (1974) School refusal, truancy and neurotic illness. *Psychological Medicine*, **4**, 416–421.

Watson, J.B. (1913) Psychology as the behaviorist views it. *Psychological Review*, **20**, 158–177.

Watson, J.B. and Rayner, R. (1920) Conditioned emotional reactions. *Journal of Experimental Psychology*, **3**, 1–14.

Wolpe, J. (1958) *Psychotherapy by Reciprocal Inhibition*. Stanford University Press, Stanford, CA.

Young, J.E. (1994) *Cognitive Therapy for Personality Disorders: A Schema-focused Approach*, revised edition. Practitioner's Resource Series. Professional Resource Press, Sarasota, FL.

FURTHER READING

Beck, J. (1995) *Cognitive Therapy: Basics and Beyond*. Guilford Press, New York.

Ellis, A. (1962) *Reason and Emotion in Psychotherapy*. Stuart, New York.

Guidano, V.F. and Liotti, G. (1983) *Cognitive Processes and Emotional Disorders: A Structural Approach to Psychotherapy*. Guilford Press, New York.

Hawton, K., Salkovskis, P.M., Kirk, J. and Clark, D.M. (eds) (1989) *Cognitive Behaviour Therapy for Psychiatric Problems: A Practical Guide*. Oxford Medical, Oxford.

5

THE SOCIAL MODEL

'We do not look out for any particular organ as the seat of insanity, nor do we pretend to operate directly on the mind or soul, but we aim to study the patient as a unity, as an individuum in all his physical, intellectual, moral and social relations.'

H. van Leeuwen (Dutch psychiatrist), 1854

All social models in psychiatry have the same fundamental premise. They regard the wider influence of social forces as more important than other factors as causes or precipitants of mental illness. At a superficial level the social model appears to be a simple extension of the psychodynamic model. Whereas the dynamic model sees the patient in the context of his personal relationships, particularly those within the family, the social model sees him as a player on a much larger stage, that of society as a whole. But this implies that the methods of the psychodynamic model will be equally appropriate for the social one. This is not true as there are other important differences between the models that are summarized in Table 5.1 and explored in more detail below.

CENTRAL TENETS OF THE SOCIAL MODEL

- Mental disorder is often triggered by life events that appear to be independent
- Social forces linked to class, occupational status and social role are the precipitants of mental disorder
- People with mental disorder often become and remain disordered because of societal influences
- Much of apparent mental disorder is falsely labelled as illness when it should be regarded as temporary maladjustment

---

Models for Mental Disorder: Conceptual Models in Psychiatry, Fifth Edition. Peter Tyrer.
© 2013 John Wiley & Sons, Ltd. Published 2013 by John Wiley & Sons, Ltd.

Table 5.1:   Main differences between social and psychodynamic models

	Psychodynamic model	Social model
Causes of disorder	Personal, highly specific, and not immediately understandable	Based on general theories of groups, communities and cultures
Precipitants of disorder	Unconscious mental mechanisms	Observed environmental factors explain onset of illness
Symptoms	Have symbolic significance based on past childhood conflict	Determined by nature of social event
Treatment	Personal or group psychotherapy	Treated by social and environmental adjustment
Status of patient	Seen as ill and requiring therapy	Seen as a normal reaction to specific circumstances

Sociology and psychiatry have long enjoyed healthy collaboration, and the social psychiatry model of mental illness has developed from this. Perhaps

Emil Durkheim should be regarded as the founding member of the social psychiatry school. In his classical work on suicide in 1897 he showed that social factors, particularly isolation and its accompanying loss of social bonds and restraints (anomie), were important in predicting suicide and, indeed, in many instances appeared to be direct causes. The realization that mental illness was a direct consequence of social forces took time to take root as most psychiatrists of the day were followers of Kraepelin (disease model) or Freud (psychodynamic model) (Giddens, 1972). The disease model was convinced that a physical explanation of psychiatric illness was just around the corner, and the psychodynamic model was busy looking beyond the obvious to the obscure but with the same aim, to find a common 'illness' explanation for mental disorder. In the past 50 years the shortcomings of the other models have led to serious consideration and, more recently, acceptance of the social model. In particular there has been a growing body of evidence that social forces are primary in the cause and persistence of much of mental illness (e.g. Brown and Harris, 1978; Totman, 1979; Ritscher *et al.*, 2001) and now the social model can stand unsupported.

In some ways it is surprising that it has taken so long for the social model to reach respectability in psychiatry. For years man has looked on many forms of illness as reactions to external events. For centuries people have been said to die 'from a broken heart' following the loss of a spouse. This has sometimes been regarded as an old wives' tale but it is true; after bereavement there is a higher risk of death in a spouse in the succeeding six months and heart disease is the commonest cause of death in this time (Parkes *et al.*, 1967).

LIFE EVENTS, SOCIAL FORCES AND ENDOGENOUS ILLNESSES

Where social psychologists and psychiatrists have made particular advances recently is in measuring the impact of social forces using acceptable scientific criteria. We know there are many social forces that can impinge on an individual but they vary greatly in degree and nature, and some may be a consequence rather than a cause of illness. Merely describing them is not enough for hypotheses to be tested; they have to be quantified. Many mental disorders were originally thought to be completely independent of social or environmental factors and when an illness became manifest it was governed by acts of God or the movement of the planets and stars (followers of astrology will note that this is still an active proposition). One of the common names for those who show mental illness is 'lunatic', which literally means 'moonstruck', as the exhibition of mental disorder was thought to vary depending on the phases of the moon, with the time of full moon being of particular risk. Although many lay people and health professionals still believe this to be true there is no evidence in its favour (Owen *et al.*, 1998).

The much more obvious suggestion that social factors and forces were involved in the creation of mental illness has taken longer than it should have done to become properly rooted. An important stimulus to the importance of these factors came from studies of life events – the formal description of key events in people's lives that have a major impact. Holmes and Rahe were the first to introduce the concept of giving scores to different life events. Their scale, the Social Readjustment Rating Scale (Holmes and Rahe, 1967), was the first of many that have become increasingly sophisticated (e.g. Paykel *et al.*, 1971; Brown and Harris, 1978). Holmes and Rahe quantified the severity of a particular life event by the degree of change it produces, and all events were recorded as life change units (LCU). The relative values of LCUs were determined by giving the scale of 42 items to 400 healthy people and asking them to record the amount of readjustment that each event would require. Although this may seem an idiosyncratic personal view a surprising degree of agreement was reached. All events carry an LCU score. An event such as bereavement scores 100 LCUs and one such as moving house scores only 20 LCUs. Further development of this and similar scales has separated events that are independent of illness from those which might be associated with it. For example, a person with an attack of bronchitis would often feel ill for a few days before developing chest symptoms and therefore not go to work. This does not mean that failure to go to work is a social cause of bronchitis. On the other hand, if a person gets abnormally depressed two weeks after his house is burgled, it is likely that the burglary was an important factor in the development of his depression as it is an independent event.

To varying degrees, life events have been shown to be important in the causation of mental illness. They are extremely important in common mental disorders such as anxiety and depression and mixtures of the two, cothymia (Tyrer, 2001). It has been shown that such events are seven times greater in patients with these disorders than in matched control subjects (Cooper and Sylph, 1973). This perhaps is so well known that it does not need repeating. Major upheavals in our lives are stressful and stress and mental illness often go together. The anxiety of the newly appointed business executive trying to keep to the schedules demanded by his company, the depression of a mother with young children who is deserted by her husband, the hypochondriasis of the nuclear power worker exposed to radiation, the impotence of a young man immediately following his marriage; they are all reactions which are immediately understandable in the context of life events and it would be foolish to consider the problems in isolation. We are all prone to mental disturbance when unpleasant events strike us without warning and 'stress reactions' are the most common mental disorders.

The major work of George Brown and his colleagues has also showed that whether life events have major or minor impact depends greatly on the context in which they occur, and can have particularly long-lasting effects when they occur in childhood (Brown, 2002). These events and their social circumstances also have a major effect on the way in which people respond to other forms of treatment that claim that they are independent. Thus a person with depression who is treated with antidepressants according to the biological model, may have their clinical response determined much more by their social circumstances than by their medication (Brown *et al.*, 2010).

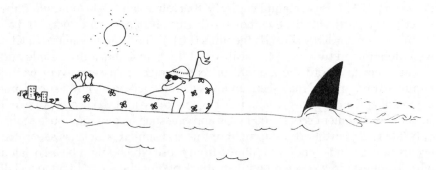

'We are all prone to mental disturbance when unpleasant events strike us without warning . . .'

Severe mental illness used to be thought of in a different light, but the influence of the social model has been enormous in changing perceptions.

The adjective 'endogenous' used to be commonly used to indicate that such illness is independent of external (or 'exogenous') circumstances. So in the past major classification of depression was into two groups, endogenous and reactive. For the former it was thought there was an internal clock within the individual which predetermined when the episode of illness would start and the timing, and indeed the course, could not be altered in any way. We now know this to be wrong, and the more recent classifications of depression merely separate them by the adjectives, mild, moderate and severe. Schizophrenia used to be thought of as an illness that was independent of social factors. Its original name, dementia praecox (precocious dementia), illustrates this. But there is now abundant evidence that there are significantly more independent life events immediately before the onset of schizophrenia compared with a control population (Brown and Birley, 1968) and that future relapse is not only dependent on life events (Vaughn and Leff, 1973), but also on the level of emotion expressed by others that the patient experiences after leaving hospital.

If there is a high level of critical emotion expressed then the patient is much more likely to relapse than if exposed to a calmer emotional context. It may therefore be preferable for a schizophrenic patient to return to a place that is relatively under-stimulated (e.g. a lodging house) after leaving hospital, instead of to the bosom of his family, where he may not be able to cope with the emotional pressures. There are also more life events immediately before the onset of severe depression (Paykel *et al.*, 1969) and mania (Ambelas, 1979), conditions which in the past were also thought to be 'endogenous'.

Work on depressed patients has shown that certain social factors are commonly found in such patients. Women living in a London borough were chosen at random and interviewed using a diagnostic schedule. The group diagnosed as depressed were found to have more young children at home, less full-time or part-time employment, and fewer confidants with whom to discuss their worries than the non-depressed group (Brown and Harris, 1978). An interesting difference was found between the social factors in 'neurotic' and 'endogenous' depression. The time between major life changes (particularly those involving loss) and the depression was significantly greater for 'endogenously' depressed patients. Thus the apparently unpredictable onset of endogenous depression may be misleading; social factors are important but, because those that are responsible may have been experienced many months or years before the depression begins, they are missed. The interval between the onset of the precipitating social factors and the depression alters the form of the eventual illness so the clinical features of 'endogenous' and 'neurotic/reactive' depression differ.

IDENTIFICATION OF SOCIAL CAUSES OF MENTAL ILLNESS

It is not particularly difficult to identify the social factors that are responsible for mental illness. In fact, it is almost too easy, because the causes are so prominent that they may often be ignored by the investigator as too obvious. For example, studies of alcoholism (often euphemistically called drinking problems) were carried out many years ago to determine the type of person most at risk. Many thought that the alcoholic was born with an abnormal form of metabolism that led to a greater risk of addiction. It is now known that the obvious precipitating factors, the availability and price of alcoholic drinks, followed by the consumption, are also the main causes of alcoholism. In countries where the price of alcohol is very high or the outlets to the public are strictly controlled there is a significantly lower incidence of alcoholism than in other countries, such as France and Italy, in which regular alcohol consumption is part of daily life.

There is now excellent evidence that severe mental illness is more common in those who come from socially deprived backgrounds. It used to be thought that the major reason for this was the social drift of ill people towards poor urban areas, after a famous study carried out in Chicago 75 years ago (Faris and Dunham, 1939). However, those who live in these deprived areas for most of their lives also have higher rates of severe mental illness and the mental health needs of a population are best predicted by its social deprivation index (Jarman *et al.*, 1992).

SOCIAL MODEL IN PRACTICE

As with the previous two models it is worth while studying a problem commonly seen in clinical practice to illustrate the value of the social model and its differing standpoint from other models.

CASE HISTORY

Presenting problem

A man aged 24 is seen in a general hospital following a suicide attempt. He had taken an overdose of sleeping tablets after a fairly trivial row with his girlfriend. He is referred to the psychiatrist because he repeatedly expresses the view that life is hopeless and that there is nothing to live for.

History of disorder

Eighteen months ago he was made redundant from his job as an engineer. This was devastating for him as he had done an engineering apprenticeship and thought that with this training he would have a job for life. Unfortunately, his company had shifted its interest towards microcomputers and no longer needed his skills.

Interpretation: His depression is understandable in the context of his life circumstances; it is normal to feel depressed after such a devastating blow to your ambitions and self-esteem.

He was now living on unemployment benefit which was less than half his original wage. With this income he was unable to save any money and was not able to obtain a mortgage to buy a house. He had hoped to raise sufficient cash for a down-payment on a house before getting married, but recently his relationship with his girlfriend had begun to deteriorate. They were having repeated arguments, mainly about money, and on the night of the overdose she had threatened to leave him.

Interpretation: The young man has suffered two important losses for which he could not be held responsible. He has suffered loss of income because he was made redundant and loss of self-respect because he does not see himself as a useful member of society. Social forces have made him depressed but he is not really ill. He has an adjustment reaction to the loss of his job.

Treatment

The doctor who saw the young man was a supporter of the social model and decided not to follow the path of conventional psychiatry and 'admit to hospital for further observation'. Instead he arranged for the man to join a day hospital group of young people who had been similarly disempowered by social circumstances beyond their control.

Interpretation: Admission to hospital would reinforce feelings of alienation and uselessness: showing him there are others with similar problems who are getting better could restore hope.

Following further treatment, linked to work-training schemes in which he received token payment, he improved further and he and his girlfriend were reconciled. Subsequently he obtained a new job as a computer engineer and developed a new career.

Interpretation: The return to a working environment promotes self-esteem and respect from others through his attitude and behaviour, and this is worth a thousand externally administered therapies.

CAUSES AND SYMPTOMS OF MENTAL ILLNESS WITH THE SOCIAL MODEL

The psychodynamic model emphasizes that symptoms are not what they seem and serve as a means of distracting the therapist from the real cause of mental conflict. The social model maintains that mental illness is related clearly to social factors and there is no difficulty in predicting that one will follow from the other, as for example with the higher rates of consultation in inner cities. There is also some evidence that the immediate 'built environment', the houses and streets where people live, can have an effect on their mental health (Weich *et al.*, 2002).

It is also useful to look further and see whether the causes have any links with certain types of mental disorder. In general these links are present. For example, it has been shown that depression is not just related to additional life events but is especially associated with events that are constructed as loss. This can be the loss of a close relative or another person, of material possessions such as a house or car, or something more abstract such as an ideal, ambition or belief. Thus depression is preceded by many more 'exit' events than 'entrance' ones (Paykel *et al.*, 1969). Similarly, there is evidence that anxiety, which is essentially a symptom implying threat or danger, is more likely to be preceded by events signifying danger or threat than depressive symptoms, and that mixed feelings of anxiety and depression are associated with mixed events signifying threat and loss (Finlay-Jones and Brown, 1981).

To return to the case of the young man who has taken an overdose, it is easy to see the relationship between the cause and symptoms of his depression. Until recently he was making good progress in his job and had a settled future. Since then he has lost his job, has been unable to raise sufficient money as a down-payment on his house, and on the night of the overdose was threatened with an even greater loss, that of his girlfriend. In telling the psychiatrist about his feelings he comes back repeatedly to the notion that he has given up trying to solve his problems. He maintains that all his attempts to overcome his employment, financial and personal problems are doomed to fail as each solution seems to be replaced by a greater problem. This phenomenon of 'giving up' often marks the dividing line between illness and health. An important part of treatment will be to help him find alternative ways of recovering his self-esteem.

The reader will see that there is a much simpler relationship between the causes and symptoms in the social model compared with the psychodynamic model. According to the psychotherapist most symptoms are false clues and only explained through symbolism, but in the social model they are directly related, and, what is more, easily seen to be related, to the cause of the symptoms. They are also more closely related in time than with the psycho-dynamic model. The causes of the symptoms are usually to be found within the recent past with the social model whereas one invokes unconscious conflict in childhood more frequently in the dynamic model.

Because the social model sees the individual in the setting of society it does not have fixed ideas of what constitutes psychiatric illness. The disease, psychodynamic and cognitive-behavioural models all look to an internal explanation of psychiatric illness that stands on its own. The social model is concerned that the labelling of psychiatric illness may create its own disorder, as once labelled as ill a person may feel he has to act the part. There is a view, exemplified in its most exaggerated form by the writings of Thomas Szasz (1961), that mental illness is not real illness but only a label that doctors place on patients when they deviate from the norm. It is perfectly legitimate for a patient to consult the doctor for help if he or she feels unwell but it is inappropriate for the doctor to act on behalf of society and give any form of treatment against the person's will. Because there are no objective tests for mental illness the doctor has no authority to carry out this type of treatment and it only succeeds in practice because the doctor and patient play their respective roles with enthusiasm. Although Szasz's view goes rather further than most advocates of the social model, it demonstrates the importance of society in determining attitudes and opinions about mental illness.

ALLOWING ADJUSTMENT TO TAKE PLACE IN ADVERSITY

One advantage of the social model is that it does not force treatment on those who are perceived as mentally ill. Often it is only necessary to acknowledge that there is a temporary loss of function created by adversity that will soon be corrected, and then normal service will be resumed. Mental illness remains a stigmatized subject and the less a person's life is disrupted when temporarily ill, the better.

Often such illness is better treated in more traditional settings. A villager near the Victoria Falls in Zimbabwe in Africa who is perceived to have some form of mental illness (*penga*) is as likely to consult his local witch doctor (*nganga*) as a Western-trained doctor or psychiatrist. This is because the cause of mental illness is thought most commonly to be due to evil spirits (*ngosi*) rather than the more common Western explanations dotted elsewhere throughout this book. We do not have randomized controlled trials of the effect of the *ngangas'* interventions – designed to drive out the *ngosi* – compared with more typical Western models, but the continued popularity of *ngangas* suggests that they are continuing to impress by their results. When we collected herbal remedies from *ngangas* many years ago as part of a university expedition we found some powerful, but toxic, compounds; fortunately these were all denatured and nullified by boiling and other treatments before being given to patients. The effect of these remedies was therefore no more, but no less, than giving a placebo.

The social model would predict this. The important element here is that the visit to the *nganga* is a socially acceptable and 'normalizing' one – it allows some acknowledgement of illness in the cultural setting, so that the patient and others realize that all is not as usual, but also strengthens the bonds between all concerned and allows a period of rest and partial function before a return to normality. The *nganga* may choose to involve a whole community in driving away the evil spirits and gives important roles to different people. This type of treatment has been going on for centuries, so who says the multidisciplinary team is a new idea?

Contrast this with a similar problem in a Western affluent society. The young man will interpret his symptoms differently because of his cultural background. When he presents these to others he is recognized by his family and the rest of society as ill and medical help is requested. Instead of a *nganga* in tribal headdress he sees a more prosaic figure, the general practitioner, who asks for a psychiatrist to visit. The psychiatric, in turn, makes a diagnosis and may recommend admission to hospital. If the young man refuses he is likely to be admitted compulsorily so it is unwise for him to argue.

DEALING WITH DEVIANCE IN SOCIETY

It would be wrong to compare the rights and wrongs of each system of assessment and management of disorders in different settings, but the examples above illustrate how much of mental symptomatology depends on cultural background and the accepted norms of society. To take another example, in the former USSR society learned to respect the State and convention decreed that open criticism was normally considered unwise. Those who not only criticized it but did so publicly were highly unusual people. They knew it was an offence against the State punishable by law and there was no immediate benefit in making the criticism. The authorities responded frequently by replacing law with medicine. Psychiatrists were called to see the dissident (in Western eyes), or deviant (in Eastern ones), as he or she must be abnormal to make such heinous allegations. A suitable diagnosis was found, the most common being 'sluggish schizophrenia', and treatment in a psychiatric hospital, sometimes for several years, was arranged (Bloch and Reddaway, 1980).

It is worth looking at the concept of sluggish schizophrenia in more detail as it shows all the disadvantages of the biological model of mental illness. The concept, introduced by Andrei Snezhnevsky (1968), is an apparently respectable way of separating positive and negative symptoms of schizophrenia, but it became diverted to a more sinister purpose. Although the exact figures will probably never be known, according to Robert van Voren (2010), up to a third of all political prisoners in the Soviet Union at the height of the Cold

War were detained in psychiatric hospitals with the diagnosis of sluggish schizophrenia. The advantage of sluggish schizophrenia in this context was that it was a very elastic diagnosis. According to Smulevich (1989) it was 'an independent diagnostic category characterized by a slowly progressive course, subclinical manifestations in the latent period, overt psychopathological symptoms in the active period, and then by a gradual reduction of positive symptoms, with negative symptoms predominating the clinical picture during patient stabilization'. Any intelligent reader can see from this description that, once you have stripped away the jargon, virtually anybody could be diagnosed with this disorder at some stage of its development, and when the terminology for the diagnosis implied that anyone who deviated from the norm could have the condition, it is easy to see that political dissidents would satisfy all the diagnostic criteria.

Fortunately, things have changed. I was at a meeting in Serbia in 2012 in which an esteemed Russian psychiatrist, Valery Krasnov, presented some figures showing the proportion of patients detained with sluggish schizophrenia in Russian psychiatric hospitals. The proportion had fallen from over 25% in the early 1980s to less than 2% by 2004. When the diagnosis of a condition changes as much as this even the Russian psychiatric system acknowledged, at least implicitly as Dr Krasnov let the figures speak for themselves, that something must have been wrong.

In the United Kingdom most people criticize the State at some time or another; it is often a sign of political maturity to do so. We therefore shudder in horror at the thought that some people are regarded as mad if they act in the same way in another country. But we should not be too complacent. Society determines what is acceptable and this cannot be exported to a different society. Have you noticed, for example, that attacks on, and threats to, politicians are treated as acceptable or dealt with according to the normal process of law, whereas similar action taken against members of our Royal Family is more likely to lead to admission to a psychiatric hospital. Are anti-royalists madder than other protesters? Or is it something to do with the rules of society?

So clearly there is a need for society to have doctors and patients and, accordingly, to set up roles for each of them. First of all, society sets up rules by which some problems are classified as suitable to be dealt with by law and others are regarded as mental illness. Doctors are appointed with interest and expertise in mental health (really mental ill-health). Although, like all doctors, their first duty is to the patient's welfare they also have a duty to society. Although doctors like to convince themselves that they always thinks of the patient first, in practice society's needs always win. In 1938 Patrick Hamilton wrote a play called *Gaslight*. The plot concerns the admission of a woman against her will to a mental hospital. She is no longer wanted by her husband and various tricks are played on her in an attempt to make out she is mentally ill. There is a family history of mental disturbance and her husband plays on this, making out to the medical authorities that his wife has also become mentally disturbed. By securing her admission to mental hospital he is free to go off with another woman. Throughout the play we are left in no doubt that the unfortunate victim is continuously sane.

This is not a fanciful idea. The '*Gaslight* phenomenon', as it has been named, is now described in the psychiatric literature (Barton and Whitehead, 1969; Smith and Sinanan, 1972; Lund and Gardiner, 1977), and is now so pervasive that it is no longer worthy of published record. When people deviate from the accepted norms of behaviour they are often labelled 'mad' because this leads to a suitable mode of disposal. No-one questions the motives of society; all is subservient to the scrutiny of the patient and his so-called abnormalities. If society, whether in the form of its smallest unit, the family, or its largest, the community, perceives the patient as a nuisance, the wheels of control are set in motion and institutional care is arranged. It is very difficult to reverse this process and all doctors working in psychiatric hospitals know many patients who have no significant mental disturbance but stay in hospital because they have nowhere else go.

Psychiatrists used to be the only doctors with the power to take away people's liberty. They still have that power, and now that responsibility can be devolved to other mental health professionals under the New Mental Health Act of 2009. Deprivation of liberty is an exceptional power and society is a little wary of those who possess it. For this reason it is important for the public to think of psychiatrists as rather strange but non-threatening figures, who talk vaguely and largely incomprehensibly. It suits society to label most psychiatrists as advocates of the psychodynamic model, as these odd people in search of the id are harmless cranks and seem far removed from the machinery of state. But in fact, all psychiatrists are in a sense agents of the State unless they practise privately, or in specialties such as psychotherapy where these issues are largely avoided as the patients are much more likely to be well.

The advocate of the social model may feel it necessary to go beyond helping his patients to understand how society influences and perpetuates psychological distress. They may also feel it necessary to try and alter the way society deals with the mentally ill by changing social attitudes. A single-minded social psychiatrist in Italy, Franco Basaglia, did just this. He came to regard psychiatric hospitals as instruments of 'social violence' that led to patients being excluded from normal society. The answer was to close the mental hospitals. After dramatically reducing the in-patient population of the San

Giovanni mental hospital in Trieste in northern Italy from 1200 to 350 patients in eight years he started a political movement that became so influential that the government was forced to act. A law was passed in 1978 which forbade the admission of any new patients to mental hospitals and arranged instead for them to be seen at special psychiatric admission units in general hospitals.

Basaglia died in 1982 but his work goes on. Although the reform has been criticized (Jones *et al.*, 1991), it has now been accepted. Indeed, in an influential review of the Italian experience, Tansella and Williams (1987) conclude that 'in places where the reform has been properly implemented, the Italian model of community care without mental hospitals is able to cope with the problems presented by the whole range of psychiatric patients resident in a catchment area'. The Italians have reminded us forcefully that all psychiatry has socio-political overtones and unless we are fully in tune with the social model we will go astray.

The social model reminds us that all symptoms and behaviour have to be considered in the context of the society from which they emanate. This will not only mould and modify the mental abnormalities but also determine the boundary line between normal and abnormal. We must be careful not to pretend that there is some independent objective criterion of mental disorder that is unaffected by these external factors. Our relationship with other people is heavily dependent on social factors although we would prefer not to admit it to ourselves. There are many who can give accounts along the lines of the police officer who hails a taxi on behalf of a drunk and delinquent toff in a smart suit, and yet immediately afterwards calls in reinforcements to deal with a homeless drunk who is arrested for breach of the peace. Doctors can also be affected by this and diagnose the former as 'social drinking' and the latter as 'alcohol dependence'.

USING THE SOCIAL MODEL TO REVERSE DIAGNOSTIC PRACTICE

We have seen already that the social model has helped to reverse diagnostic practice in Russia, a classic example of society needing to change rather than the individual with alleged mental illness. A classical example of this that is closer to home is the 'mental disease' called homosexuality. Long treatises were written about this allegedly severe mental illness and its causes in the late nineteenth and early twentieth centuries. The foremost authority on the subject, Richard von Krafft-Ebing, considered that the disease was created early in utero by 'inversion of the brain'. Now all this is seen as nonsense in the more mature countries of the world, but unfortunately not in all. In no diagnostic system is homosexuality regarded as a disease. This is because society has changed and become much more inclusive. There are still battles to be won, as everyone will know who looks at the recent controversy in the Church of England, but, by and large, people are becoming tolerant and more understanding of what used to be called deviance and which is now recognized to be part of the spectrum of normal existence.

By seeing a psychiatric patient as a temporarily misplaced unit in society the social model avoids the tendency to ascribe illness, inherent in other models. The aim is to help the individual to take up an acceptable role again, not to correct a biochemical disturbance, exorcize an unresolved conflict or recondition behaviour. In many instances it will be realized quickly that the person being seen for help is not really unwell at all and is just in the wrong place at the wrong time, as it was 100 years ago if you were homosexual.

NIDOTHERAPY

But many forms of mental illness need much more than mere acceptance as their presence causes suffering and hardship. Even with the advances of drug and psychological treatments in the past 50 years, the simple and sad fact is that a large number of people with mental illness do not show significant improvement, or respond only partly to treatment and relapse afterwards. The social model has an answer to this – it is called 'nidotherapy'. Nidotherapy describes the systematic manipulation of the environment to accommodate the requirements of those with persistent mental illness (Tyrer, 2002; Tyrer et al., 2003) and is particularly suited to the social model. 'Nidotherapy' derives from the Latin word, nidus, a nest, as, when you think about it, a bird's nest is an ideal example of an environment that is perfectly adapted to an object that is placed within it, as it can adjust its shape at will to achieve a perfect fit. For those who never seem to fit in because of their mental health difficulties, and this includes many with chronic depression, obsessions, autistic spectrum disorders, some types of schizophrenia and personality disorders, there often seems to be no treatment that helps and no place where the person feels satisfied and content.

For these people, nidotherapy may be the answer. It makes no attempt to treat the patient directly and instead, in a collaborative exercise, involves the patient and therapist in a systematic examination of all parts of the environment, physical, social and personal, to see what might be changed to make a better fit. The aim is not to change the person but to improve general function and well-being. Targets for environmental change are agreed, sometimes with the help of an independent arbiter if patient and therapist cannot always agree, and attempts made to introduce them over an agreed realistic timescale

(Tyrer and Bajaj, 2005, 2012; Tyrer, 2009). Thus society, in its broadest sense, by allowing its health professionals to make societal changes to accommodate patients' needs, is providing a solution.

Nidotherapy is still an experimental treatment and in some ways it is best not described as a treatment at all since it is not focused on the patient but on the environment. But we think it can be called treatment because it involves the patient closely in deciding what environment is needed. When little in the way of medical therapy was available environmental solutions were often adopted. Bed rest, a quiet holiday in the country, a visit to a spa, and a sojourn in a sanatorium high in the mountains, are all environmental solutions for such problems, most of which had very little in the way of an evidence base. These solutions were decided by doctors, often with very little discussion of their benefits in handicaps, and in nidotherapy it is considered essential to bring the patient with you in deciding which environments would be the most suitable.

Nidotherapy is also an important component of what is called the recovery model in psychiatry. This is discussed in more detail in Chapter 6 but it emphasizes the collaborative role of patient and therapist in coming together to find solutions to difficult long-term problems that primarily involve environmental change.

We also must be careful not to get snarled up in jargon. Most of us use the principles of nidotherapy time after time again in our daily lives. At school we study subjects we are good at, and those we hope will lead to occupations where we feel most valued and successful. We look for partners with whom we feel affinity, support and love; this helps to buttress us against all the troubles that are thrown at us in a busy and confusing world. If we have the choice we choose to live in a house, or flat or other accommodation that we like and which is conveniently situated. In each task, and I think they really are tasks even though they often appear to be done quite smoothly, we are making environmental choices. The physical, occupational, social, geographical and personal environments all link together in this context. I doubt whether anyone reading this book could deny that at times they have felt extremely uncomfortable, if not unhappy, in certain places or at certain times in their past, and in correcting this unhappiness the choice was made, not to take some form of treatment – this would normally be considered anathema – but to change the environment and so bring your mood back to normal. Nidotherapy is a treatment that constitutes a formal extension of this to change the environments of people who have really become so stuck in a jungle of competing awfulness that they can see no way to turn and have no-one to help them. The nidotherapist is there to act as a guide to get out of this jungle and start afresh.

OTHER APPLICATIONS OF THE SOCIAL MODEL

Family therapy (Barker, 1981) has been an important development in psychiatry. While developed to a large extent by psychodynamic psychiatrists, it was also pioneered by social and anthropological scientists, and is closely related conceptually to these fields. The family approach takes the family as the key social group, and regards the family system as powerfully influential in allotting and maintaining social roles. Part of fitting in to the environment is to make sure these roles are appropriate ones and sometimes a family's views have to be challenged and specialized help given in creating the scope for change. The social model is particularly keen to avoid one of these roles, that of becoming a dependent patient unnecessarily. Unfortunately, as the skills of life become more specialized it becomes more difficult to acquire them, particularly if you have been out of circulation, as it were, acquiring a different set of roles in a psychiatric unit.

Life is a drama and to succeed you need to have acting skills. Many lack the social skills that are necessary for them to fill the role for which they are chosen. We all have to appear confident and in control at times when we have no idea what we are doing, and to talk freely when we do not feel like saying a word. We also have to appear to people in a way that reflects our competence and abilities. Unfortunately many people, and this includes so many psychiatric patients, lack these abilities or have spent too long speaking their minds without fear of contradiction because they are perceived to have an affliction. This is particularly likely to happen after prolonged institutional care.

Nevertheless, many of those who seem to have permanent handicaps have the ability to change and indeed to act completely different roles. One example of this has been tried in our own hospital, where with the aid of our music therapists we have been able to mount concerts in which patients play and sing the roles of staff and vice versa, and before long nobody is quite sure which is which. When this has extended to involving a patient who has spent six years in hospital under almost continuous compulsory orders in taking one of the key parts in a special concert performance at the Annual Meeting of the Royal College of Psychiatrists, we can only guess at the limits of their versatility.

SUMMARY

The social model takes a broader view of psychiatric disorder than any other model. It takes the person with apparent mental disorder and studies their problems in the round, not as odd diagnostic shapes that need to be fitted into appropriately designed boxes. Mental illness, more than any other form of illness, involves close interaction with others, and unless we take into account all the aspects of the environment we fail as practitioners. To use the analogy of a man looking down a microscope to study an illness: the disease, psychodynamic and cognitive-behavioural models are all concerned with microscopic details of structure, dynamic change and activity in the moving parts. The patient is being studied closely but in isolation. By contrast, in the social model, not only is the patient being studied under the microscope, but also the doctor, those employing the doctor, and the society that sets up the system that allows people to be examined in this way. The social model is truly a big comprehensive model and deserves our respect and full support.

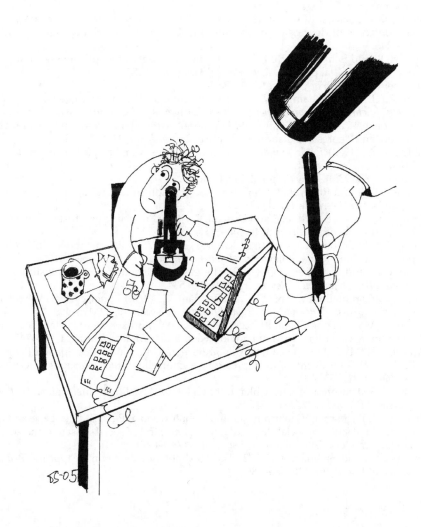

REFERENCES

Ambelas, A. (1979) Psychologically stressful events in the precipitation of manic episodes. *British Journal of Psychiatry*, **135**, 15–21.

Barker, P. (1981) *Basic Family Therapy*. Granada, London.

Barton, R. and Whitehead, T.A. (1969) The gaslight phenomenon. *Lancet*, **i**, 1258–1260.

Bloch, S. and Reddaway, P. (1980) *Russia's Political Hospitals: Abuse of Psychiatry in the Soviet Union*. Gollancz, London.

Brown, G.W. (2002) Measurement and the epidemiology of childhood trauma. *Seminars in Clinical Neuropsychiatry*, **7**, 66–79.

Brown, G.W. and Birley, J.L.T. (1968) Crises and life events and the onset of schizophrenia. *Journal of Health and Social Behaviour*, **9**, 203–214.

Brown, G. and Harris, T. (1978) *The Social Origins of Depression*. Tavistock Publications, London.

Brown, G.W., Harris, T.O., Kendrick, T., *et al.* (2010) Antidepressants, social adversity and outcome of depression in general practice. *Journal of Affective Disorders*, **121**, 239–246.

Cooper, B. and Sylph, J. (1973) Life events and the onset of neurotic illness: an investigation in general practice. *Psychological Medicine*, **3**, 421–435.

Durkheim, E. (1897) *Le Suicide*. Alcan, Paris.

Faris, R.E.L. and Dunham, H.W. (1939) *Mental Disorders in Urban Areas: An Ecological Study of Schizophrenia and Other Psychoses*. University of Chicago Press, Chicago.

Finlay-Jones, R. and Brown, G.W. (1981) Types of stressful life events and the onset of anxiety and depressive disorders. *Psychological Medicine*, **11**, 803–815.

Giddens, A. (1972) *Emile Durkheim; Selected Writings*. Cambridge University Press, London.

Hamilton, P. (1938) *Gaslight*. Constable, London.

Holmes, T.H. and Rahe, R.H. (1967) The social readjustment rating scale. *Journal of Psychosomatic Research*, **11**, 213–218.

Jarman, B., Hirsch, S., White, P. and Driscoll, R. (1992) Predicting psychiatric admission rates. *British Medical Journal*, **304**, 1146–1151.

Jones, K., Wilkinson, G. and Craig, T.K. (1991) The 1978 Italian mental health law – a personal evaluation: a review. *British Journal of Psychiatry*, **159**, 556–561.

Lund, C.K. and Gardiner, A.Q. (1977) The gaslight phenomenon – an institutional variant. *British Journal of Psychiatry*, **131**, 533–534.

Owen, C., Tarantello, C., Jones, M. and Tennant, C. (1998) Lunar cycles and violent behaviour. *Australian and New Zealand Journal of Psychiatry*, **32**, 496–499.

Parkes, C.M., Benjamin, B. and Fitzgerald, R.G. (1967) Broken heart: a statistical survey of increased mortality among widowers. *British Medical Journal*, **1**, 740–743.

Paykel, E.S., Myers, J.K., Diendelt, M.N., Klerman, G.L., Lindenthal, J.J. and Pepper, M.P. (1969) Life events and depression: a controlled study. *Archives of General Psychiatry*, **21**, 753–760.

Paykel, E.S., Prusoff, B.A. and Uhlenhuth, E.H. (1971) Scaling of life events. *Archives of General Psychiatry*, **25**, 340–347.

Ritscher, J.E.B., Warner, V., Johnson, J.G. and Dohrenwend, B.P. (2001) Inter-generational longitudinal study of social class and depression: a test of social causation and social selection models. *British Journal of Psychiatry*, **178**, 84–90.

Smith, C.G. and Sinanan, K. (1972) The 'gaslight phenomenon' reappears. *British Journal of Psychiatry*, **120**, 685–686.

Smulevich, A.B. (1989) Sluggish schizophrenia in the modern classification of mental illness. *Schizophrenia Bulletin*, **15**, 533–539.

Snezhnevsky, A.V. (1968) The symptomatology, clinical forms and nosology of schizophrenia. In: J.G. Howells (ed.) *Modern Perspectives in World Psychiatry*, pp 425–447. Oliver and Boyd, Edinburgh.

Szasz, T.S. (1961) *The Myth of Mental Illness*. Harper and Row, New York.

Tansella, M. and Williams, P. (1987) The Italian experience and its implications. *Psychological Medicine*, **17**, 283–289.

Totman, R. (1979) *Social Causes of Illness*. Souvenir Press, London.

Tyrer, P. (2001) The case for cothymia: mixed anxiety and depression as a single diagnosis. *British Journal of Psychiatry*, **179**, 191–193.

Tyrer, P. (2002) Nidotherapy: a new approach to the treatment of personality disorder. *Acta Psychiatrica Scandinavica*, **105**, 469–471.

Tyrer, P. (2009) *Nidotherapy: Harmonising the Environment with the Patient*. RCPsych Press, London.

Tyrer, P. and Bajaj, P. (2005) Nidotherapy: making the environment do the therapeutic work. *Advances in Psychiatric Treatment*, **11**, 232–238.

Tyrer, P., Sensky, T. and Mitchard, S. (2003) The principles of nidotherapy in the treatment of persistent mental and personality disorders. *Psychotherapy and Psychosomatics*, **72**, 350–356.

Van Voren, R. (2010) Political abuse of psychiatry – an historical overview. *Schizophrenia Bulletin*, **36**, 33–35.

Vaughn, C.E. and Leff, J.P. (1973) The influence of family and social factors on the course of psychiatric illness: a comparison of schizophrenic and depressed neurotic outpatients. *British Journal of Psychiatry*, **129**, 125–137.

Weich, S., Blanchard, M., Price, M., Burton, E., Erens, B. and Sproston, K. (2002) Mental health and the built environment: cross-sectional survey of individual and contextual risk factors for depression. *British Journal of Psychiatry*, **180**, 428–433.

FURTHER READING

Tyrer, P. (2009) *Nidotherapy: Harmonising the Environment with the Patient*. RCPsych Press, London.

6

AN INTEGRATED MODEL

In our unfolding beauty contest displayed in previous pages the four models have presented their attributes in their best light. In the words of the dodo after the end of the caucus race in *Alice in Wonderland*, 'everybody has won, and all must have prizes'. The disease model would no doubt get the Alzheimer's prize for the best vital statistics linking brain and body, the psychodynamic model would get the prize for the greatest sex appeal, particularly for those parts needing dynamic exploration that the camera

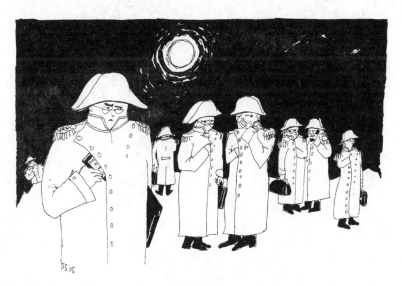

'Nothing would be more alarming than for all psychiatrists to think in the same way'

Models for Mental Disorder: Conceptual Models in Psychiatry, Fifth Edition. Peter Tyrer.
© 2013 John Wiley & Sons, Ltd. Published 2013 by John Wiley & Sons, Ltd.

could not reach, the cognitive-behavioural model would win the Thinking Man's Crumpet award for logical and delightful construction at all levels, and the social model would win the Germaine Greer Female Eunuch award for getting over the real message of beauty contests to the world. However, it takes all sorts, as they say, and nothing would be more alarming than for all psychiatrists to think in the same way.

How can we reconcile these different models to the practice of mental health care? What we can say, without much fear of contradiction, is that practitioners are generally more comfortable with some models than others, and this is predictable through their preferred treatment decisions. In general, biologically orientated (white-coated) psychiatrists prefer the disease

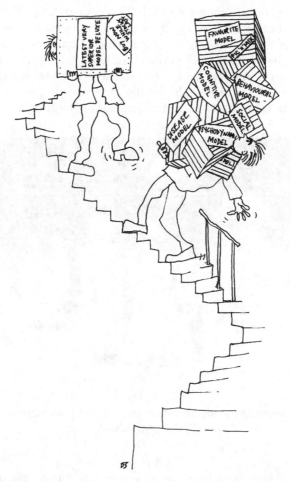

'. . . will bend over backwards to say that they are eclectic . . .'

model, the (open-necked, polo-necked) psychotherapist prefers the psychodynamic model, the efficient 'scientist practitioner' (Salkovskis, 2002) prefers the cognitive-behavioural model, and the (blue-jeaned and open-sandalled) social worker prefers the social model. You can ignore the sartorial connections if you wish; they are merely the manifestations of common prejudices.

However, if you challenge each of these professionals directly, they will bend over backwards to say that they are eclectic, that they use several models at different times and that they are prepared to use these flexibly to suit the circumstances. We do not deny that they intend to use these models in this way, but in practice very few do; and when you find someone who adheres absolutely to one model, such as the well-known psychologist, the late Hans Eysenck, did to the behavioural one, it is only achieved by abstinence from actual clinical contact. When exposed at the coal-face of clinical practice, single models just do not work.

A source of confusion in trying to understand psychiatry and construct models of the subject is the notion that there is an underlying psyche, or mind, which can be diagnosed, treated and cured. Of course the concept of mind is useful, but mainly in the healthy sense, and in mental illness its complexities are more to the fore. In Figure 6.1 the interrelationships between the different levels of function are illustrated. This is just as complex and ambiguous as many world events and is best conceived as an interplay between various organizational levels.

For example, let us consider the problems of a young man with an intellectual handicap due to brain injury at birth. What is 'wrong' with him, a necessary description before effective care can be given, could be described in terms of 1–4 in Figure 6.1:

1 Damaged neural connections
2 Problems in learning
3 Low self-esteem
4 Conflict between his abilities and those imposed by normal social expectations.

The 'lesion' may be a neurological one, linked clearly to the disease model, but the management involves far more than a knowledge of pathophysiology; training, understanding of functioning at more than one level, family attitudes and individual feelings are all part of the strategy of treatment. Similarly, a young woman with a social phobia (now called social anxiety) may appear to have a straightforward problem involving social behaviour and psychological perception, but at various times it can be aggravated by biochemical factors

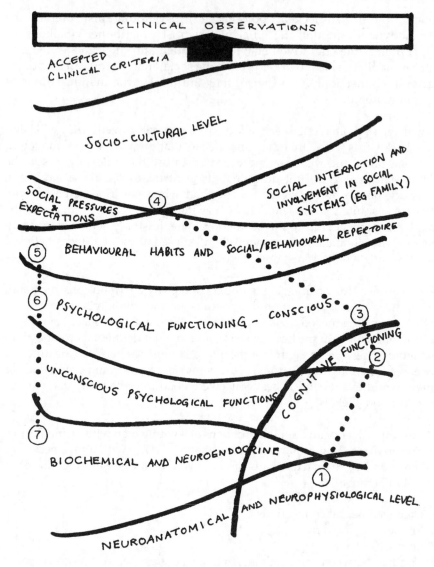

Figure 6.1:   Levels of functioning.

affecting her general mood (e.g. premenstrual exacerbation of symptoms and enhancement by concurrent depression) (5, 6 and 7 in Figure 6.1). Nevertheless, most practitioners feel comfortable with one of the four models we have described and attempt, like Procrustes (the celebrated robber in Greek legend who used to ensure his victims fitted the length of his bed by either stretching them or chopping off their legs), to fit their patients' problems to their favourite model wherever possible. It is only when this does not work that they will look elsewhere and, somewhat reluctantly, apply other models.

This is particularly evident when there is a multidisciplinary review of a difficult clinical problem. Each practitioner slants the discussion in favour of his or her preferred model and a power struggle develops. It may not appear to be a power struggle because everybody uses reasoned argument but when the outcomes seem to favour one model repeatedly it is clear that something else is going on. The approach chosen is usually that preferred by the dominant figure in the discussion and, to some extent, the others tend to go away dissatisfied. It would be wrong to say that this is a common outcome of attempts at multidisciplinary working in psychiatry. There is a genuine wish to reach consensus but each member, not always consciously, is fighting the corner of one model against the others.

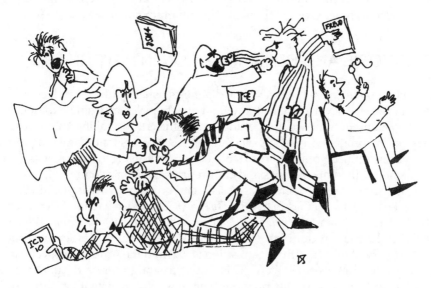

'The approach chosen is usually that preferred by the dominant figure in the discussion . . .'

In fact, it is not especially difficult to achieve consensus at some level and probably all at such discussions, including the patient, would agree the following:

1 Every patient needing mental health care is a biological entity with biochemical, pathophysiological, pharmacological and, sometimes, anatomical changes occurring because of their mental state abnormality.

2 Their disorder has important social and environmental associations; the people concerned are emotional beings who have many feelings expressed and unexpressed which often seem to be in conflict.
3 Those who suffer from mental distress have distressing thoughts and behaviour that are maladaptive. Their thinking is awry in at least some respects.
4 The extent to which they suffer is dependent on the attitudes and reactions of families and society in a wider context.

In deciding which model to use we first of all need to have a common procedure to place an individual's problem at the appropriate model. We then match treatment and other forms of management with that model, often bringing into operation the approaches of other models where necessary. A common procedure is that of diagnosis, a discipline which tends to be confined to medical members of the psychiatric team but is increasingly being recognized as necessary for all mental health practitioners.

DIAGNOSIS AND CLASSIFICATION IN PSYCHIATRY

In general medicine and surgery one diagnosis usually suffices; indeed some teachers advise never to make more than one. In psychiatry single diagnoses are less common, but we are getting more efficient in making them. It is a mark of the progress made in psychiatry in recent years that many diagnoses have been refined to such an extent that an increasing number of people throughout different countries and cultures can agree on a common language to describe mental disorders. Diagnosis is embodied in two classification systems, the *International Classification of Disease (ICD)*, which had its 10th revision (ICD-10) recently, and the *Diagnostic and Statistical Manual for Mental Disorders (DSM)*, which is in its fourth revision (DSM-IV). These classifications are published by the World Health Organization (1992) and the American Psychiatric Association (1994) respectively. This is not a straightforward subject and anyone who has read the previous chapters will realize that the word 'diagnosis' has some practitioners purring and others close to apoplexy.

Nonetheless, the proper use of classification is central to an integrated model of mental illness, but it is a dangerous business and is very unwise to enter it without a proper guide. If you are in the UK you will be most familiar with the *International Classification of Diseases (ICD)* and in the United States (and many other countries as it has spread widely) with the *Diagnostic and Statistical Manual of Mental Disorders (DSM)*. These have progressed through many different revisions since their introduction; *DSM-5* has just been published in May 2013 and *ICD-11* will be published in 2015. The official world classification of all diseases is *ICD* but, in psychiatry, *DSM* has more or less taken over gradually in most countries of the world since 1980, when the third revision was carried out under an extremely energetic and persuasive psychiatrist called Robert Spitzer. Before 1980 no-one could agree on psychiatric classification. There were many loose descriptions, frequent options to diagnose 'other' when a diagnosis did not seem to fit, and tremendous variation between different countries of the world. A classic example was the comparison of the diagnosis of schizophrenia between the USA (New York) and the UK (London) in the diagnosis of schizophrenia. When researchers showed the same case histories in videotaped form to psychiatrists in the USA and the UK there was more than a 30% discrepancy between British and American psychiatrists, which was even stronger in those working in academic departments. It may be an oversimplification but the much higher rates of schizophrenia diagnosed by American psychiatrists seemed to be a consequence of psychoanalytical orientation. If someone used odd expressions, or whose thinking was deemed to be 'woolly', they were readily diagnosed as schizophrenic in New York but not in London (Cooper *et al.*, 1972).

American psychiatry, as befits a go-ahead and vibrant country, is always ready to accept new ideas and this may explain a lot of the variation between US and British psychiatry over the years (Canada is an exception as it still has strong British roots in its thinking). So whenever a new, exciting way of looking at mental illness has crossed the Atlantic it has been embraced with enthusiasm. By contrast, the British experience has been very different. We are a pragmatic and slightly cynical nation, who look at all new ideas askance at the first instance, and demand a much greater degree of evidence and experience before we accept any new system, and then it has to be in operation for many years before we take it seriously.

This is relevant to the classification system. *DSM* in its first and second versions was hardly ever used by psychiatrists. There was no attempt to measure agreement between different diagnoses and at that time (1940s–1960s) psychoanalysis reigned more or less supreme except in a few isolated enclaves. As the psychodynamic approach (Chapter 3) could never be quite sure what the problem was before treatment had begun, not least as the concept of the unconscious meant that many aspects were hidden, the notion of diagnosing patients on the basis of one interview was hardly popular and could be criticized strongly as premature.

As psychoanalysis was replaced by a more scientific psychiatry the concept of diagnostic reliability, the measure of agreement between people looking at exactly the same patients, became much more important. Robert Spitzer and others, particularly what became called the St Louis School of psychiatry under Eli Robins, concentrated those on the notion of inter-rater and temporal reliability in diagnosis. This was an understandable change. If psychiatrists cannot agree on a diagnosis no-one will take them seriously. (Even when they do agree they are not always taken seriously; in one famous high profile murder case in the UK the judge commented, after three psychiatrists had all agreed on the diagnosis, 'this is such an unusual occurrence that I am not sure if it is correct and I will take the opposite view'. He ordered the patient concerned to be detained in prison rather than a special hospital as a consequence. Inter-rater reliability describes the level of agreement at the same point in time; temporal reliability describes the level of agreement over the course of time. The St Louis School argued cogently that if a diagnosis changed frequently over a short period it could hardly be a good diagnosis, and therefore temporal reliability needed to be good unless the diagnosis was clearly a short-term one.

DSM-III was published in 1980 and immediately became a great success. What Robert Spitzer had done was very clever. He invited a large number of experts to meetings to discuss different diagnostic concepts and they managed to come to general agreement. How? Alix Spiegel (2005) has described the process delightfully: 'There was just one problem with this utopian vision of better psychiatry through science: the "science" hadn't yet been done.'

'There was very little systematic research, and much of the research that existed was really a hodgepodge – scattered, inconsistent, and ambiguous,' Theodore Millon, one of the members of the *DSM-III* task force, says. 'I think the majority of us recognized that the amount of good, solid science upon which we were making our decisions was pretty modest.'

Members of the various committees would regularly meet and attempt to come up with more specific and comprehensive descriptions of mental disorders. David Shaffer, a British psychiatrist who worked on the *DSM-III* and the *DSM-III-R*, told me that the sessions were often chaotic. 'There would be these meetings of the so-called experts or advisers, and people would be standing and sitting and moving around,' he said. 'People would talk on top of each other. But Bob would be too busy typing notes to chair the meeting in an orderly way.' One participant said that the haphazardness of the meetings he attended could be 'disquieting'. He went on, 'Suddenly, these things would happen and there didn't seem to be much basis for it except that someone just decided all of a sudden to run with it.' Allen Frances agrees that the loudest voices usually won out. Both he and Shaffer say, however, that the process designed by Spitzer was generally sound. 'There was not another way of doing it, no extensive literature that one could turn to,' Frances says. According to him, after the meetings Spitzer would retreat to his office to make sense of the information he'd collected. 'The way it worked was that after a period of erosion, with different opinions being condensed in his mind, a list of criteria would come up,' Frances says. 'It would usually be some combination of the accepted wisdom of the group, as interpreted by Bob, with a little added weight to the people he respected most, and a little bit to whoever got there last.'

Because there are very few records of the process, it is hard to pin down exactly how Spitzer and his staff determined which mental disorders to include in the new manual and which to reject. Spitzer seems to have made many of the final decisions with minimal consultation. 'He must have had some internal criteria,' Shaffer says. 'But I don't always know what they were.' One afternoon in his office at Columbia, I asked Spitzer what factors would lead him to add a new disease. 'How logical it was,' he said, vaguely. 'Whether it fits in. The main thing was that it had to make sense. It had to be logical.' He went on, 'For most of the categories, it was just the best thinking of people who seemed to have expertise in the area.'

(Alix Spiegel, 2005)

So here is diagnosis in 1980. It is not much better in 2013, despite attempts to get a diagnosis based on biomarkers and other objective measures of mental illness (the disease model has not done well here). There are two important messages of *DSM-III* that have influenced all further revisions – (i) a reliable diagnosis is better than an unreliable diagnosis, and (ii) an agreed reliable diagnosis cannot be regarded as a valid one unless it is supported by additional evidence. Unfortunately the second message was forgotten and *DSM-III* became the bible of psychiatry in many people's eyes. In fact 'the bible' is quite a good metaphor because there are many ways of interpreting it. One group regards it as next to perfect, and if these are followed properly by all residents in psychiatry we will have a unified diagnostic system that leads to better treatment and much better outcomes. Another group feels the *DSM* is a very good system for diagnosing Americans with mental illness in the north-eastern seaboard of the USA but not nearly as good diagnosing illnesses elsewhere, and try very hard to find culturally acceptable equivalents – the many translations and modifications of the Bible over the course of centuries give support to this approach. Then there are many other ways of interpreting the Bible that allow much more flexibility in its interpretation. Those that support the *International Classification of Disease* classification could be included here. Finally we have the agnostics and atheists, who do not believe that the *DSM* has any bearing on real psychiatric classification and would like to abolish it altogether. Indeed, there is an organization in the UK, Campaign to Abolish Psychiatric Diagnosis (CAPSID), that exists precisely for this purpose. These are joined by other groups who are generally against psychiatry, such as the Scientologists, who use the limited credibility of all psychiatric classification systems to proclaim that psychiatrists are not proper scientists or doctors and have no place in the care of the mentally ill. The agnostics have been in powerful voice recently. I could put myself in this group at times and in my '100 words' in the *British Journal of Psychiatry* I have summarized DSM as:

'*DSM* is an American classification system that has dominated since 1980. It is disliked by many for reducing diagnostic skills to a cold list of operational criteria, yet embraced by researchers believing that it represents the first whiff of sense in an area of primitive dogma. It has almost foundered by confusing reliability with validity but the authors seem to recognize its errors and are hoping for rebirth in its 5th revision due in May 2013. The initials do not stand for Diagnosis as a Source of Money or Diagnosis for Simple Minds but the possibility of confusion is present.'

(Tyrer, 2012)

This may be slightly unfair, but there is absolutely no doubt that the *DSM* classification is much easier to use for psychiatrists than the exercise of good clinical judgement, and there is obvious concern that 'the tick box mentality' created by a set of allegedly 'operational criteria' to little more checklists is a major concern to psychiatric teachers, and that the *DSM* publications contribute a massive proportion of the funding to the American Psychiatric Association, who naturally promote it for all they are worth.

In a recent review of *DSM* process Blashfield and Fuller (1996) quoted one of the early members of the Robert Spitzer group, Jean Endicott, who paraphrased Mao Tse-Tsung, 'Let a thousand flowers bloom, even if a few of them are weeds'. But Blashfield and Fuller now counsel the opposite, 'scientists should reverse this process until the difficult but crucial task of sorting out which of the existing categories of mental disorders represent valid diagnostic concepts. Eliminating the weeds will be a challenging task (p.7)'.

In the integrated model diagnosis has to be taken into account in some way, but in doing this we have to recognize that it is very much a 'system under construction' and needs a great deal more before it can be regarded in any way as respectable. Most psychiatric disorders do not have clean diagnostic descriptions, but this does not mean that diagnosis is a waste of time. Diagnoses are useful because they allow mental health professionals and research workers to know what each is talking about so that each has a common frame of reference and because they are useful shorthand for groups of disorders which share the same clinical features, and have similar outcomes and agreed treatments. Without diagnosis in some form, people communicating with each other about different disorders are like a group from different nations, who each can only speak one language not shared by any of the others. Communicating then by sign language is open to tremendous misinterpretation.

The main diagnoses in the 10th revision of the *International Classification of Diseases (ICD-10)* are shown in Table 6.1. In admitting that most of these are probably wrong – and indeed will be superseded by the 11th revision very shortly – and nonetheless show both the value and handicaps of diagnosis.

Table 6.1: Summary of Chapter 5 of the 10th revision of the *International Classification of Diseases*

Main category	Sub-categories	Main features
Organic (F0)	Dementias Delirium Mental disorders due to physical disease Personality or behaviour disorder due to brain disease or injury	Conditions in which brain dysfunction is present, and manifested by disturbances of cognition, mood, perception or behaviour
Psychoactive substance use (F1)	States of intoxication, harmful use, dependence and withdrawal states, and psychosis resulting from use of alcohol, opioids, cannabis, sedatives, cocaine, tobacco, hallucinogens and other drugs	Includes all mental disorders which are considered to be a direct consequence of drug use and which would not have occurred without consumption of the drug (or drugs)
Schizophrenia, schizotypal and delusional disorders (F2)	Schizophrenia Schizotypal disorder Persistent delusional disorders Acute and transient psychotic disorders Schizoaffective disorders	Conditions in which there are distortions of thinking, perception and mood not due to an organic condition and which are most prominent in schizophrenia
Mood (affective) disorders (F3)	Manic episodes Depressive episodes Bipolar affective disorder Recurrent depressive disorder Persistent affective disorders	A range of disorders in which disturbance of mood (affect) is the main feature, together with other symptoms which are easily understood in the context of change of mood and activity
Neurotic, stress-related and somatoform disorders (F4)	Phobic disorder Other anxiety disorders Obsessive–compulsive disorder Stress and adjustment disorders Dissociative and conversion disorders Somatoform disorders	A group of disorders in which certain symptoms, historically recognized as part of 'neurosis', are most marked and which may have a psychological causation
Behavioural syndromes and mental disorders associated with physiological dysfunction and hormone imbalance (F5)	Eating disorders Psychogenic sleep disorders Sexual dysfunctions Mental disorders associated with the puerperium	Disorders in which physiological and hormonal factors may be involved in causation or be prominent in association with the disorder

Table 6.1: *continued*

Main category	Sub-categories	Main features
Disorders of adult personality and behaviour (F6)	Personality disorder Enduring personality change Habit and impulse disorders Gender identity disorders Sexual preference disorders	Conditions of clinical significance in which behaviour patterns tend to be persistent and which are 'the expression of the individual's characteristic life-style and mode of relating to self and others'
Mental retardation (F7)	Mild mental retardation Moderate mental retardation Severe mental retardation Profound mental retardation Other types of mental retardation	A condition of 'arrested or incomplete development of the mind', manifest by impairment of skills commonly associated with intelligence
Disorders of psychological development (F8)	Developmental disorders of speech and language Specific developmental disorder of scholastic skills Specific developmental disorder of motor function Pervasive developmental disorders (e.g. autism)	Conditions that begin in infancy or childhood, delay in the development of functions related to maturation of the nervous system, and which generally have a steady rather than remitting course
Behavioural and emotional disorders with onset occurring in childhood or adolescence (F9)	Hyperkinetic disorder Conduct disorder Mixed disorder of conduct and emotions Emotional disorder of childhood Disorders of social function (childhood) Tic disorders Other behavioural or emotional disorders	A mixture of disorders in which the only common features are an onset early in life and a fluctuating or unpredictable course

Taken from Chapter 5 of the 10th revision of the *International Classification of Diseases* (ICD-10), 1992. World Health Organization.

A good diagnosis carves nature at its joints so that each condition stands alone in splendid isolation from its fellows. Very few psychiatric diagnoses do this, but it does not mean they should be abandoned as useless, or regarded merely as labels that only serve to stigmatize patients and minimize the special features of each problem that make it unique. Those who criticize diagnosis and use other systems (of which perhaps the most popular are those based on problem-orientation) will realize that, although there are some advantages in their approach, there is considerable economy in transmitting information when it can be simplified to straightforward diagnostic terms.

Sometimes this can only be done by using more than one diagnosis and deciding, somewhat arbitrarily, that one should take precedence over the others. Thus from Table 6.1 it is easy to see how some patients can have diagnoses from several categories. Consider, for example, a young man whom one of us saw recently in hospital after breaking his leg following a fall when he was drunk. (The different diagnoses from *ICD-10* are indicated in italics during the description and the detailed coding also given.) He was seen shortly after he had returned from the operating theatre where he had received a general anaesthetic during the treatment of an open fracture in which full cleaning (debridement) of the wound was considered necessary because of the fear of gangrene. After recovering from the anaesthetic he was confused and disorientated and muttered nonsensical replies to questions. *Diagnosis in F0 category – delirium (05.0).* Although it was impossible to get a detailed history about his problem he admitted to heavy alcohol consumption, mainly beer, over the previous six years. Whenever he stopped drinking for more than 12 hours he developed severe stomach pains and a craving for alcohol. *Diagnosis in F1 category – alcohol dependence syndrome (10.2).* On questioning him about his reason for heavy alcohol consumption he admitted to persistent, relatively mild depression which he claimed was dulled to some extent by drinking and therefore made bearable. However, even when drunk, he still felt depressed to some extent. *Diagnosis F3 – dysthymic disorder (34.1).* He also complained that he was anxious for much of the time because he had no confidence in his dealings with other people and felt that people were scrutinizing him closely whenever he met with them. He felt very embarrassed among groups of people that he did not know and tried to avoid such groups wherever possible. *Diagnosis F4 – social phobia (40.1).* On enquiring about his background it was clear that he had been unsettled in his personal relationships ever since adolescence. He was excessively dependent on his mother and, despite several attempts to leave home, he always returned to her care. He relied excessively on her although he had confidence to go out and meet other people when he had a few drinks. *Diagnosis F6 – dependent personality disorder (60.7).* During his childhood he had been a slow developer and had been protected by his parents to a greater extent than the other two children in the family, partly because he was more anxious than the other children. He also wet his bed at night on average 5–10 times each month until the age of 12. This had been investigated in hospital without any organic cause being found. *Diagnosis F9 – non-organic enuresis (98.0).*

Each of these diagnoses has a clear description associated with diagnostic guidelines. When they have been diagnosed correctly a great deal more information is conveyed to the listener or reader who knows the detailed criteria for the diagnoses. Although it is possible to make fun of the list of diagnoses in the patient described above, if we opted for economy and listed all these diagnoses it would convey at least as much information as the long prose account above and would be much easier to collect and code. Diagnosis in psychiatry, like diagnosis in any branch of medicine, is simply a form of shorthand between informed people and, like most shorthand, it does not look pretty but is effective for communication.

Let us look at the process of diagnosis in practice. The assessment usually proceeds in three steps, two descriptive and the third explanatory. The explanatory step is not a statement of observable facts but a working hypothesis about the nature of the disorder, and this is the step where the various models for mental disorder are invoked.

Step 1

This is a simple account of the reason for referral and in literal terms is the proper use of problem-orientation (e.g. 'I can't sleep, I don't get on with people, I get no enjoyment out of life, people are persecuting me'). Sometimes the reasons for referral are much more complex, and include many more people, and in such cases it may be appropriate to ask the question, 'Who is complaining about what?' (Steinberg, 1989, 2005).

Step 2

This is to identify an accepted clinical psychiatric disorder, if there is one. Not all problems presented to the psychiatrist or mental health worker are sufficient to merit the label of a psychiatric disorder. It is not always helpful to label an unhappy or worried or misbehaving person 'depressed', 'anxious' or 'borderline' for example, unless their feelings or misbehaviour really amount to something that justifies special intervention. However, this is a very large topic that cannot be taken further here. Those who would like to pursue this ethical–philosophical point should read further (Foucault, 1967; Szasz, 1961; Lewis, 1953; and Ramon, 1985; among others).

Step 3

This is the construction of a working hypothesis about the nature of the problem. It is at this stage that we attempt, relying more on clinical experience than hard evidence, to give due weight to the various possible components

---

CASE HISTORY

Step 1

A man is referred by A&E after an overdose. He has no general practitioner. He lives alone but was taken to hospital by his landlord who thinks 'something should be done' and is anxious that there is no recurrence. His only relatives are in Scotland, and cannot be contacted.

Step 2

On examination he has depressed mood, is actively thinking about suicide, and has additional symptoms of disturbed sleep, loss of interest, loss of appetite and weight loss, and hopelessness about the future. These lead to a diagnosis of a depressive episode.

Step 3

This man has become depressed this time because of the loss of his job. He is significantly depressed at present and may require antidepressant drugs. At the same time, however, his capacity to use psychological approaches such as cognitive-behavioural therapy should be explored because these are at least as good as drug treatments and have fewer adverse effects. Whatever the usefulness of medication or psychotherapy, his social isolation and poor social skills mean that his unemployment may well become chronic, and occupational and social assessment and help will both be needed. While these are being explored, he will need close observation because his mental state, social isolation and history make him a high risk for a further suicidal attempt. The feasibility and usefulness of further discussion with his landlord, and contacting his relatives, should be explored, with appropriate permissions; and he ought to be registered with a general practitioner. This may extend to a full environmental analysis to allow him to see what needs to be changed in his life and how it might be done (the nidotherapy approach).

---

of a patient's case. One person's distress may seem to be caused and maintained by present circumstances; another by the influence of past experiences; another by the influence of their physiological state and genetic inheritance. On this basis we would have to make decisions about the sort of approach most likely to help: social help, behavioural training, individual psychotherapy, family therapy or medication.

HOW CAN DIFFERENT MODELS INTERACT?

There is no reason why the different conceptual models we have outlined should not interact with each other, and it will be seen that the general approach we are recommending includes looking for such interactions.

Thus there is a well-recognized association between blood lead levels in children and their having educational and behavioural problems – sufficient evidence, it may be said, to justify urgent measures to reduce this atmospheric pollution. However, there is also an association between educational and behavioural problems and living in poor neighbourhoods with poor schooling in inner cities with high local levels of atmospheric lead, for example, in the shadow of motorways. Here we see socio-economic (and indeed political) factors interacting with children's behavioural and educational performance and their neurophysiological status.

Yet another example is the simple behavioural model by which a patient develops a phobia for a situation in which he or she had a bad experience – perhaps a fear of flying conditioned by a near-accident. In clinical practice such clear-cut causes are unusual. What is more often seen is the development of anxiety (or other persisting distress) in a situation that to a specific individual is unusually highly disturbing. Thousands of people may have the same experience (e.g. discomfort in crowds) without developing symptoms that persist and become disabling. A few, however, develop a phobic state. Is this because some people become more highly aroused than others in crowded circumstances? Is this because some are physiologically different (i.e. more vulnerable to maladaptive learning)? Or is it because for some their emotional development gives a highly anxiety-laden personal meaning to the situation? Since not everyone responds in the same way, there is clearly a personal characteristic or set of characteristics interposed between stimulus and response. In some people this may be their physiological learning set, in others it may be unconscious determinants of what they find particularly frightening, and in others it may be determined by personality status. We see no problem in hypothesizing that both psychodynamic and physiological factors can influence the individual response to a situation, although the degree to which each operates in the individual case will vary.

THE MEDICAL MODEL

The reader may wonder how we have come so far without describing the best-known (and much maligned) model of all. We believe the term 'medical model' is widely misused and misunderstood, and in particular that it is erroneous to equate it with the disease model. As we mentioned in the introduction, we have not used this description because of confusion surrounding the adjective 'medical'. The pedigree of the 'medical model' is not to be found in the annals of discovery about the physical origins and treatment of disease, but in the nature of the doctor–patient relationship. This relationship has archetypal qualities quite distinct from other professional relationships. In it the physician purports to diagnose disorder or its absence in the patient by using particular understanding of symptoms and signs and their implications.

Other professional–client relationships are quite different. The craftsman does something for other people, whether it is putting up a shelf or designing a house. The lawyer acts as the client's advocate, putting his or her case in the best possible way, whatever its merits or demerits. The policeman stops people doing things that the law says they should not do. We would argue that a psychotherapist or social worker who identifies neurotic conflict 'in' a client and proceeds to treat this 'anomaly' is using the medical model. On the other hand a family therapist or social worker who believes that the problem is not individual disorder but lies in the family group relationships is taking a genuinely different approach.

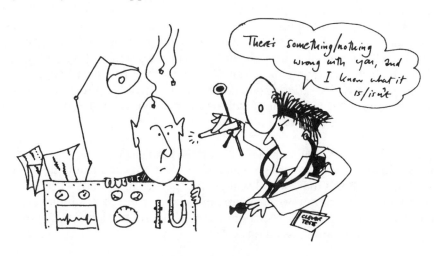

'The medical model'

The medical model, by our definition, is one in which the diagnosis of individual disorder is central, whatever the conceptual model of individual disorder used: disease model, psychodynamic model, cognitive-behavioural model or some of the social models. It is a pragmatic rather than an ideologically pure model and, annoying though this may be for purists, quite ready to ditch models of assessment and management if they do not work, and adopt or adapt methods that do. Even worse for the orthodoxies, it is prepared to use one model for diagnosis and another for treatment: thus we may believe that the nature of a patient's anxiety is best understood in psychodynamic terms, but behaviour therapy is the most effective treatment. Or, that the nature of a retarded child's major incapacity is neurophysiological, but the necessary treatment is a mixture of education, social skills training and family work – which may well include working psychodynamically with the parents' distress and disappointment.

In the following pages we describe how each of the four models described earlier in this book can be used effectively and in harmony with other models.

MATCHING MODELS TO DISORDER

Are there ways of combining these models so that they co-exist more peacefully? At first sight this may seem difficult. How can symptoms be thought of as abnormal patterns of thinking and behaviour (cognitive-behavioural model), the products of social forces (social model), smoke screens that obscure the true psychic conflict (psychodynamic model), and the building blocks of illness syndromes (disease model), all at the same time? It is true that this cannot be done for the whole range of mental disorder and distress, but you will have noticed already that each model illuminates some corners of psychiatry better than others. The disease model is particularly appropriate for the psychoses (i.e. *manic depressive illness*, schizophrenia and the organic illnesses (e.g. dementia) with psychiatric symptoms) in which identifiable disease already exists.

The psychodynamic model helps to understand aspects of both normal behaviour and symptomatology that otherwise appear meaningless. The social model shows that mentally ill people, particularly those with the less severe disorders, cannot be considered in isolation from their families, social and cultural background. The cognitive-behavioural model is at its best in explaining and treating disabling symptoms.

CENTRAL TENETS OF THE INTEGRATIVE MODEL

- We each have several levels of functioning ranging from biological functions through to personal decision-making
- When mental disorder develops it can affect one or more levels
- At different times in the course of the disorder the predominant level of dysfunction may change
- Each model in psychiatry links specifically to one level of function
- Successful treatment of mental disorders involves matching the main level of disturbance with the appropriate model and its philosophy of management

---

At another level, the cognitive-behavioural and disease models are particularly orientated towards focused treatment, and the social and psychodynamic models towards understanding the causes and motivation, although they also incorporate therapy. The different treatments in psychiatry align themselves nicely alongside the models. Physical treatment such as drug therapy, electroconvulsive therapy (ECT) and psychosurgical operations are involved with the disease model; psychotherapy with the psychodynamic model; rehabilitation, social skills training, nidotherapy and social engineering (which is part of sociology, economics and politics) with the social model; and cognitive-behavioural therapy with the cognitive-behavioural model. If the divisions were mutually exclusive there would be less conflict between the different models, but because they overlap argument begins – the psychotherapist believes the behaviourist and the 'organic' psychiatrist are missing aspects of their patients' cases, and vice versa. This is a clinical and ideological concern. When it comes to how much influence each model should have on the training curriculum there can be major arguments. For theoretical and academic purposes, it is no bad thing that each model should have its adherents, explorers and teachers. For good clinical practice, research purposes and teaching it is important that the positive features of all the models be taken seriously, because any or all may be helpful for the next patient, whoever is the therapist.

RESOLVING CONFLICTS IN THE INTEGRATED MODEL

Because most people do not yet use the integrated model there are bound to be conflicts in care, particularly in today's practice where decisions are made by multidisciplinary teams. I should like to illustrate this by describing a personal experience.

Many years ago I was treating a patient with what is now called 'hoarding disorder' in the classification systems. This describes a group of people who are compelled to collect and retain large amounts of furniture and other goods than most would regard as rubbish or garbage. As a consequence their homes become completely cluttered by belongings and acquisitions that often reduce their living space to a tiny area. This also leads to public health problems, as hygiene is usually poor and there is much opportunity for vermin to become established. There are also fire hazards when combustible material is stored in bulk.

There is no known standard treatment for hoarding disorder but it is placed within the obsessional group of disorders by many people. The big difference from other similar disorders is that people who hoard regard it as a perfectly normal activity and do not take kindly to people stopping them. My patient was a highly intelligent man who regarded himself as an eco-warrior needed to preserve the planet from unnecessary destruction and so chose to recycle almost everything that came into his life, as well as, unfortunately, many of the goods that were deposited in dustbins outside his flat. When the complaints of others, and the attention of public health officials about the risks to others in his block of flats, escalated to crisis point it became necessary to admit the patient to hospital, where valiant attempts were made to give a new diagnosis and allowed him to be given additional treatment, but almost all of this was unsuccessful.

Over the course of 10 years all the different models described in this book were attempted. Our patient attended a day hospital where both psychodynamic and supportive approaches were tried; attempts were made to integrate him into the local community via the day hospital so that he could understand the impact his hoarding had on others and adjust his life accordingly (social model), he saw a psychologist who attempted to reduce his hoarding behaviour by classical behaviour methodology, and he received antidepressants (as he was undoubtedly depressed because of this isolation and conflict with others) and also antipsychotic drugs (in the forlorn hope that this behaviour might be part of a psychotic disorder). After his third, quite long, admission it was decided to treat him with nidotherapy, as until then, every single treatment had really been given against his will. In terms of his personality, he had a treatment-resisting disorder (Tyrer *et al.*, 2003), in that he did not regard his behaviour is any way as unusual or abnormal, and really wanted his environment altered so he could carry out his hoarding undisturbed. In the course of this assessment he agreed that his hoarding might be reduced but only on condition that he was allowed to organize his flat in the way he wanted. As at this stage he was still in hospital and as his flat was a public health hazard we felt we had a way forward. Eventually we agreed that his flat could be redecorated entirely in the way that he wanted provided, of course, it did not present a hazard to himself or others.

Unfortunately this was not agreed by another worker, separate from the team, who wanted to have the flat cleaned out by the local council as this 'was the normal procedure', and matters became deadlocked. As the patient was becoming extremely frustrated by a long stay in hospital in the end our team decorated the flat to our patient's requirements at less than one tenth of the sum that the council would have charged (it all came from his savings, which were considerable, as his expenses were so limited), and the patient was discharged home shortly afterwards. Eventually he had to move as his block of flats was being demolished and now he is placed in a supported home where he still tends to hoard but this is anticipated by the staff there and never gets completely out of control.

This could seem like an excellent example of the integrated model in practice, and, indeed, I think it was. The biological, psychodynamic, cognitive behavioural and social models had been tried to varying degrees, without success, and eventually overcome by variation of the social model, nidotherapy. Using this approach, all other models can still coexist as the plan in nidotherapy is to change the environment and not the person. This indeed is what happened, his environment was changed in a rather unusual way – he insisted on magnolia skirting boards and grey walls in his flat and we painted them accordingly – and subsequently he continued to attend supportive groups and remain under the care of the community team.

Unfortunately , because I was regarded as the instigator of this deviation from normal procedure I, and other members of the team, were reported to the hospital trust concerned and an investigation was carried out into my conduct in particular, as I was regarded as the ringleader of this unusual painting event. Because no justification could be found for a clinical team painting someone's flat I was eventually reprimanded formally for the unusual offence of 'trying to do my best for the patient, but not following accepted guidelines'. Guidelines are sometimes a problem in the recommendation of treatment for mental disorders because they can stick too rigidly to a specific model. The model that others were adopting in our patient's case was that he lacked capacity to decide on the painting of his house and others had to decide on his behalf. He strongly rejected this argument, and demanded his autonomy, and we felt that the capacity argument was an excuse for taking over from the patient in a paternalistic way.

When I repeat this story to colleagues, they cannot believe that anyone could object to the plan that our team initiated. It seemed a simple solution to a problem that was especially desired by the patient and was no more than common sense in practice. Unfortunately there are many examples of practice in mental health in which common sense goes out of the window and is replaced by a set of accepted procedures that make no allowance for the individual. A good integrated model of mental illness has to incorporate the views of the person being treated at least as much, if not considerably more, than the wishes of highly trained experts in the caring team.

LEVELS OF DISTRESS AND DISORDER

It is also very important to remember that mental disorder often develops (or improves) gradually, and at different times the features of illness change. The acutely ill schizophrenic patient with delusions of his mind being controlled by an alien force may present quite a different picture five years later when he has no florid symptoms but is prevented by apathy, social withdrawal and accommodation problems from returning to the social background from which he came. It is useful to consider the different levels of illness and the extent to which they interfere with normal mental function and behaviour before we look at the application of the models. Even when a disorder does not develop chronologically in this way, some or all of what follows illustrates facets of function and malfunction in mental disorder. The levels extend from mild distress at one end, through to symptoms of behaviour change, and end with disintegration of normal function at the other extreme.

Level I: Distress

The person is aware of new mental feelings, often unpleasant, such as sadness, nervousness, tension, puzzlement, irritability and anger. These are noticed more frequently than normal, and the immediate cause is usually recognizable. For example, what is often called 'postnatal blues' comes into this category. After childbirth there are significant hormonal and other biological changes, but there is also the radical change of a demanding, vulnerable and time-consuming infant. Mothers get short of sleep from frequent nightly interruptions for feeding, stresses develop between mother and father until they adjust to the new arrival, and there are increased domestic demands at a time when quiet recuperation would be more appropriate. The mental distress usually is summed up in the ubiquitous term 'nerves' and is accepted as a transitory phenomenon. These feelings amount to emotional distress but are almost universal, and this distinguishes them from mental disorder. Similarly, the tension and stress of front-line soldiers fighting in two world wars (for example in the Great War, where the attrition of trench warfare seemed bound to produce extremes of mental distress) can be regarded as universal phenomena. In such situations it is abnormal not to feel distressed and threatened. The symptoms experienced are usually diffuse and variable and will always improve when the stressor has been removed (if they do not we see the beginnings of mental disorder as opposed to distress, as in the post-traumatic syndromes).

It is less straightforward when the stressor is an internal one. For example, the mental stresses in the early stages of schizophrenia are of a quite different nature. The sufferer is aware that something odd is going on, a stage sometimes described as 'delusional mood', but cannot be sure of the source of his feelings. He usually finds the answer in the external world in the form of a delusion. However, in the early stages of the condition his emotions are little different from those who are distressed because of external stresses.

Level 2: Symptoms

In this phase the continuing emotional conflict becomes more focused on mental and physical complaints. These sometimes become highly specific and are not so directly associated with a precipitating factor. The sufferer remains aware that his feelings or behaviour differ from normal.

In conventional terminology 'insight is maintained' (see the 'Glossary of terms' for what exactly this is meant to mean) and the person may present quite normally to the world at large because he aspires towards normal functioning and tries to compensate for his disability. At this stage, too, the symptoms do not affect behaviour significantly, so general observation reveals nothing amiss. Most of the symptoms of common mental disorder come into this stage: the fears of the agoraphobic, the constant preoccupations of the ruminating obsessional, the despair of the depressed, the preoccupations of the hypochondriac and the constant worries and panic attacks of those with anxiety are all symptomatically equivalent. Unlike the symptoms in the first stage these feelings are not explicable as universal reactions; they are shown only by a minority and occur inappropriately. Apart from these specific symptoms the sufferer functions fairly well and high mental organization is retained except for short periods during the worst symptoms. People at this stage rarely find it helps to remove an apparently precipitating cause. They carry their troubles with them, and a simple change of scene, occupation or social contact will not solve the problem.

Level 3: Irrational thinking

Once symptoms persist there is the danger that they will become reinforced by distorted thinking. As we noted in Chapter 4, depressed people who withdraw from society can easily develop the 'mental set' that no-one wants to know them, and unexplained panic attacks can be misinterpreted as symptoms of physical disease. This mode of thinking only reinforces the symptoms and so there is a danger they will persist.

Level 4: Changed behaviour – disability and problems in relationships

When the symptoms of the third stage become more severe or prolonged there are changes in behaviour. The agoraphobic individual finds that avoidance of open spaces, supermarkets and public transport is preferable to the fear that these situations arouse. Similarly, the obsessional patient finds that prolonged and repeated rituals such as hand-washing briefly relieve the tension of his constant doubts and ruminations, and the depressed person becomes socially withdrawn and refuses to meet anyone, thereby increasing his isolation and despair. The change in behaviour signals to the outside world that all is not well; a composed exterior does not then disguise the change in behaviour and social functioning. If this change is dramatic enough it can seem to replace the symptoms altogether. For example, agoraphobia, which is more common in women, can develop to the point of complete avoidance of the outside world. In this grossly socially handicapped state, the person concerned may be symptom-free.

Now someone cannot change to this degree without other people being involved too. To remain (as in this case) housebound, other members of the patient's circle, usually his or her family, make adjustments too. The decision of, say, the husband of an agoraphobic woman to 'put up with it', organize himself and the children to do the shopping, is an adjustment, and it may be reasonably asked whether this response is helpful or not.

Other forms of abnormal behaviour are also included in this stage whether or not they are associated with symptoms. This varies from such basic problems as difficulty in self-feeding by mentally handicapped children to more complex actions such as persistent truanting or repeated acts of self-injury. The behaviour is considered to be abnormal because it is counterproductive or even damaging – it does not solve the problem in any way and may even make it worse. You will notice that this stage differs from the earlier ones in that the patient is not necessarily seeking help because of unpleasant feelings. Abnormal behaviour may not be regarded as abnormal by the person showing it, and other people – 'society' – may be the chief instigators in trying to alter the behaviour, a common situation in attitudes to personality disorders. This introduces an ethical aspect of management which does not necessarily apply in the earlier stages.

Thus we see that when behaviour is out of the ordinary, for whatever reason, social functioning and relationships, from the closest family matters to more remote cultural and social expectations, are usually impaired in several ways.

Level 5: Disintegration

In the earlier stages the person is capable of a wide range of normal function outside a specific area of malfunction or handicap. At the fifth level of mental disorder this boundary is reduced or even removed. The abnormality is so major that it can affect all mental activity. Thinking, feelings and behaviour are all affected and the personality appears to undergo dramatic changes. The imprecise term, psychosis, is usually used for disorders of this degree. Although it is imprecise it is now recognized to be a pretty good collective term, and the old split between manic-depressive (bipolar) disorder and schizophrenia is much less certain than it used to be (Craddock and Owen, 2005). As mental function becomes globally disordered, personal awareness of illness is often lost as well. Because of this absence of insight, treatment without the patient's permission is sometimes needed, and this introduces ethical issues. Because the person's view of the world is no longer determined by reality, he develops false beliefs (delusions), incorrect perceptions (illusions and hallucinations), and may feel he no longer has any control over his own mental function, which seems to have passed to an outside agency (passivity feelings and delusions of control). Such features may develop in part from the person's attempt to rationalize the irrational. If the world does not make sense there has to be an internal restructuring to give it some sort of order, although this tends to become one which other people cannot share.

In the face of such disorganization all semblance of integrated function disappears. Normal contact through speech and non-verbal communication becomes impossible, important drives such as hunger, thirst and sex become deranged, and hospital admission is often necessary as much to safeguard general health and protect other people as to treat the disorder. When patients with this degree of disorder recover and their view of reality returns to normal they are often unable to remember how they felt when they were ill. This is not surprising, as to reconcile the different perspectives of major illness and good health would require remarkable ingenuity. Perhaps this illustrates best the important qualitative difference between this degree of disorder and the other three: here the psychological experiences are in a different dimension from those of normal experience, neurotic symptoms, cognitive errors and behavioural change.

STAGES IN THE DEVELOPMENT OF MENTAL DISORDER

Obviously there is overlap between the levels of disorder described above, and they cannot be regarded as rigid categories. They are not at the same level as formal diagnoses, and during the course of a single illness any combination of the five may be seen. Let us take, for example, the course of severe depression in a married woman (Mrs X) following the death of her husband. Immediately following the loss she goes through a mourning process which is often socially ritualized, the ritual depending on her cultural background. This may last a few days to several weeks or months. In the first stage the immediate cause of the depressive symptoms is obvious, and if normal grieving can take place amidst a caring group of friends and relatives a healthy adjustment can be made to the loss. If normal grieving is arrested or inhibited, she moves into the second, symptomatic stage, when feelings of depression continue to gnaw inwardly, even though by the mechanisms of repression and denial she appears to have adjusted well to the loss and may be complimented on how well she has coped. Indeed a balance between confronting and repressing feelings may be part of healthy adjustment to loss.

If she develops a cycle of negative automatic thinking, believing she is partly to blame for her husband's death or that she is just a burden on others, she enters the third stage. Later still, social withdrawal and avoidance could lead her into the fourth stage. Attempts to adjust to the loss appear to cease altogether and other people are unable to alter her move towards isolation. Finally she develops a depressive psychosis, with delusions of poverty, unworthiness and guilt, accompanied by paranoid ideas and auditory hallucinations of an unpleasant critical kind. These tell her she is useless and that suicide is the only way out of the burden she is causing to her friends and relatives. At this stage she no longer feels ill but wicked. The characteristic bodily changes of severe depression, including marked loss of weight and appetite, constipation, sleep disturbance with waking in the early hours, and a worsening of her depressed mood with feelings of complete hopelessness and worthlessness are present. As she feels such a burden on everyone and with such low self-esteem it is not surprising that she now contemplates suicide. Meanwhile, she elicits a range of reactions from other people: sympathy, anxiety, sadness, anger and mixed feelings too.

Other disorders may only show obvious evidence of one of these phases, others two or three, but in all instances there is the possibility that the disorder can present at any of the five levels. How can this be explained?

Hierarchy of models

We are all aware of hierarchies in our lives. We all have to deal with much larger amounts of information than our brains can cope with and we order these in a way that makes this manageable. In addition to our own internal hierarchies we have external ones, most obvious in the structures of large organizations. Typically the bottom level of the organization contains the most people and the top level the fewest. A general feature of a hierarchy is that those on higher levels incorporate the characteristics of the lower levels. Thus the chairman of a large international company is regarded as representing the company at all levels. If, for example, there is a major scandal involving a functioning of the lowest level of the organization the chairman may be regarded as responsible and forced to resign even though he had no direct knowledge of the circumstances and personnel involved in the scandal.

Models in psychiatry have a similar hierarchical structure and this is shown in Figure 6.2. (We have joined together the cognitive and behavioural models in this edition of our book, but in this section it is useful to keep them separated.) The most minor mental disturbance (e.g. feeling angry and upset after failing a job interview) does not qualify for any diagnostic label but certainly creates social dysfunction and involves the social model. However, when specific symptoms are established at the second level of the hierarchy the psychodynamic model may be used. When maladaptive thinking predominates, the cognitive model is most appropriate and if the abnormality shows mainly in behaviour,

Disease model
Behavioural model
Cognitive model
Psychodynamic model
Social model

Figure 6.2: A hierarchy of models. Note that this is a true hierarchy in which each higher level comprises its own level and the features of all lower levels

Disease model (antidepressants and/or ECT to treat psychotic symptoms)
Behavioural model (reward outgoing social behaviour)
Cognitive model (encourage rational thinking)
Psychodynamic model (facilitate expression of feelings and promote adjustment)
Social model (support and care following death of husband)

Figure 6.3: Matching models with treatment in Mrs X

the behavioural model applies. The hierarchy leads directly to an appropriate programme of treatment, which can incorporate treatment from the same level as the model together with treatment beneath it (Figure 6.3).

Matching levels and models

It might have been noticed that the models of mental disorder discussed in earlier chapters match these levels of illness in many respects. The hierarchical model indicates that for each stage of psychiatric disorder there is an appropriate model whose application is only correct for that level of disorder. When the disorder moves to a different level, another model (or more than one) is applicable. The level of disorder corresponds with the model used.

At the first level of illness, which only comprises minor changes at the level of feelings, formal psychiatric attention is rarely needed, and the social model is appropriate. When specific symptoms are established in the second level the psychodynamic model may be used. When maladaptive behaviour-responses and dysfunctional thinking are present the third and fourth levels apply. This leaves the disease model which should be reserved for the severe manifestations of the fifth level.

However, this cannot be taken too rigidly. Because the different levels can all be shown at different times in the course of an illness the therapist cannot presume that any one model is suitable for a particular disorder. Nevertheless, because some disorders predominantly are expressed at one level there will be a tendency for one model to predominate. We also have to acknowledge that when all models seem to fail – as with the hoarding patient described earlier – there is nothing to be lost by adapting any of the models to fit the patient's needs.

In our introduction we emphasized that models are only of use if they fit the facts closely and provide a coherent basis for intervention, and this is part of the philosophy of evidence-based medicine. They are practical instruments rather than theoretical abstractions. To test whether this particular combination of models has any value we need to see whether our new correlative model is consistent with good psychiatric practice and whether it has any predictive value.

Fifth level: disease model

To return to our depressed patient, does our model help us to understand and treat her problem (Figure 6.3)? Most psychiatrists would see this patient at the fifth level, when her psychotic symptoms are established and admission to hospital is often necessary because of the danger of successful suicide. It does not require a great deal of skill and intellect to appreciate that the depressive illness is in some way due to the bereavement, but at this stage the underlying cause is not of immediate concern. The doctor is faced with a woman who is a suicidal risk, and possibly at risk of physical ill-health because of poor nutrition and inadequate self-care. The patient is firmly placed in the sick role, not because she is acting sick, but because she is sick. Her mental function is unbalanced because of the severity of her symptoms and decisions about treatment may have to be made independently without necessarily having the patient's cooperation. Admission to hospital and treatment with ECT and antidepressant drugs may therefore have to be given without her permission (something that could never be contemplated at a lower level in the hierarchy). During this disease phase of treatment the hospital setting and attitudes of other patients, medical and nursing staff are largely immaterial, although they will become very important as recovery progresses and should not be ignored now.

Fourth and third levels: cognitive-behavioural model

As the patient's psychotic symptoms improve, the negative thinking behind the depression will become more prominent. Feelings of guilt, blaming herself for her husband's death and believing that she cannot live without him are inappropriate assumptions that will prolong the depression. The depression must be prevented from returning to its former cognitive 'set' in which all possibility of improvement is excluded and morbid thinking preoccupies her brain. At a fairly simple level, and certainly not requiring any special skills of a cognitive therapist, staff on the ward can explore the patient's feelings and beliefs in a gentle way that helps her to understand that she can adjust to the death of her husband without being a traitor to his memory.

As the patient responds to treatment she will lose her delusions and hallucinations but remain socially withdrawn. She will probably be reluctant to eat regularly and wish to spend most of her time alone. During this time there is a danger that ruminating about her husband will again lead to a return of severe depressive symptoms. The nursing staff react to this withdrawal by encouraging more outgoing behaviour and trying to reduce the amount of time she spends ruminating on her own. These are, in effect, forms of operant conditioning. The staff will also encourage her to eat with other patients, talk to her socially instead of merely formally discussing her symptoms, and praise her when she achieves small advances such as baking cakes for other patients in the occupational therapy department or takes part in group activities on the ward.

Second level: psychodynamic model

As she improves in confidence and can face society again she will move towards the second level. This is the time to explore her thoughts and feelings about her dead husband, knowing that at first this may be a painful process. By 'working through' her loss again she can undergo the normal grieving process and restructure her world in a satisfactory and healthy way. It is likely that this stage could be carried out at a day hospital or in an outpatient clinic after discharge from in-patient care. A psychotherapist may even see her at this stage or at least see the staff concerned at separate supervision sessions so that this process can continue smoothly.

First level: social model

The first level of disorder may well become relevant after she has left hospital and is being followed up as an out-patient or under the care of a community-based team. Although she has adjusted in many ways to the loss of her husband, she cannot help being reminded of him as she sits in the house where they have spent so many years together. Provided that the treatment at the other four levels has been completed satisfactorily, a change of accommodation, preferably to one where she has greater social contacts, is all that is necessary to complete the adjustment and treatment of her depressive illness.

When changing from one approach to another during the course of a disorder one is merely moving to a different level in the hierarchy (Figure 6.3). This is hardly a revolutionary concept but is rarely formalized. In general medicine a condition such as hypertension can be viewed similarly. At level five the important aspect is to bring the blood pressure down by drug therapy or similar medical means, but once this has been achieved the patient needs to have his individual needs and personality considered, and advice given about his lifestyle, occupational pressures and personal relationships, much of which may need to come from non-medical sources.

The hierarchical approach should also predict successfully that when the level of the disorder does not correspond then the approach will be unsuccessful. There is a popular, but now outmoded, view of schizophrenia that it is not a true illness but a natural reaction of man to the oppressive conformity of our society (often attributed to Ronald Laing who popularized it). The victim can only break out of the mould cast for him by society by apparently becoming mad in the form of schizophrenia. This serves as a vehicle to 'break through to health' and therefore, according to the hypothesis, it is best to treat the condition at the first stage of our model by altering society rather than the patient. When this theory has been put to the test the evidence is universally negative. Patients do not achieve health by passing through a schizophrenic illness. If the condition is not treated using the disease model it is likely to become persistent and chronic and to damage the personality irreparably. There is similar negative evidence that disorders in the first stage of illness can be treated by the disease stage of our model. It is of no value to treat people distressed and disadvantaged by poverty and poor housing by hospital admission and drug treatment. These changes will temporarily remove the unpleasant feelings but will not alter the underlying difficulties, and by 'medicalizing' the problem the patient may be prevented from taking action himself to change matters.

The demarcation lines are not so clearly drawn when intermediate phases are considered. For example, a severely agoraphobic patient who generally avoids all situations outside the home may be treated according to level three along behavioural lines. Gradual exposure to the feared situation or prevention of conditioned avoidance by remaining in the feared situation until anxiety is resolved may be successful, but sometimes fails because of continued anxiety and panic.

In the worst form of the disorder the patient has a 'pan-phobia' of everything and can be said to reach the fifth stage of the model. It is therefore appropriate to give drug treatment to reduce or suppress the panic feelings that are interfering with behaviour therapy. Similarly, a phobic patient who is responding to behaviour therapy may need cognitive therapy to prevent him from developing any new symptoms of anxiety by further phobic avoidance, and he may also need psychotherapeutic intervention to illustrate how the disorder has been manipulated (not necessarily consciously) by either the patient or close relatives for a variety of reasons. Unless this is resolved the phobias may return.

The patient's perspective

In matching the approach of each model to treatment we have only recently become properly aware that the key person to be involved in the decision-making is usually the patient. When disintegration has occurred and capacity is absent then others have to act on the patient's behalf, but this only applies to a small proportion of those who have mental disorder. For most others, the ability to take part in decision-making over treatment is intact.

It is worth reminding ourselves what mental capacity constitutes. It has five basic elements:

- Every adult has the right to make his or her own decisions and must be assumed to have capacity to make them unless it is proved otherwise.
- A person must be given all practicable help before anyone treats them as not being able to make their own decisions.
- Just because an individual makes what might be seen as an unwise decision, they should not be treated as lacking capacity to make that decision.
- Anything done or any decision made on behalf of a person who lacks capacity must be done in their best interests.
- Anything done for or on behalf of a person who lacks capacity should be the least restrictive of their basic rights and freedoms.

All too often in practice health professionals forget about the first of these, and then misread the second and third. One of the worrying developments in the 26 years since the first edition of this book was published, is the growing number of patients who are subject to overt coercion, mainly in the form of involuntary (i.e. compulsory) admission, and also, in a more covert way, persuaded to do things they do not want to do, officially called leverage. In the laid-back sleepy country called the Netherlands we have come to expect great tolerance to deviance in all its forms, but compulsory admission has increased greatly in the past 30 years (Mulder *et al.*, 2008), and in the UK, approximately one in three of all patients in mental health care has experienced leverage (Burns *et al.*, 2011).

There are many possible reasons for this, of which perhaps the most important is the increasing risk aversion of daily life, but excessive adherence to models of care that predispose to coercion (e.g., the disease model), is probably one of the significant ones. The patient about whom I was reported to my hospital for inappropriate practice, was such an involuntary patient when we started practising nidotherapy. He had been kept in hospital, unnecessarily in my opinion, for over three months while attempts were made to clean his flat in a way that was completely counter to his wishes. Under these circumstances it is very easy for people to say that the patient 'lacks capacity', as it then gives others the opportunity to do anything they please on the grounds that it is in the patient's 'best interests'. The simple fact is that the patient should normally be in the centre of the integrated model and if he or she does not agree with what is being practised. This should be listened to loud and clear and not suppressed spuriously on grounds of impaired capacity or paternalistic concern.

This applies across all areas of mental health. We are increasingly training well-skilled practitioners who know how to administer a range of treatments because they have been 'properly trained'. I recently had a discussion with a psychologist who had been so trained in cognitive-behavioural therapy and was generally competent. This is how the conversation ran:

ME: 'How is that patient with depression that I referred recently for CBT?'

PSYCHOLOGIST: 'Unfortunately, he has not responded to treatment and I have discharged him.'

ME: 'Oh, how did that come about?'

PSYCHOLOGIST: 'I don't really understand. I gave all the treatment perfectly and he made no response of any sort; I'm sure it was the right treatment.'

ME: 'How can you say that you gave all the treatment perfectly?'

PSYCHOLOGIST: 'Well, as far as I am concerned I did give it perfectly, and I discussed it with my supervisor who agreed with me.'

ME: 'Did you ask the patient what he felt about the treatment?'

PSYCHOLOGIST: 'Yes. Of course I explained the principles of treatment at the beginning and he fully understood these.'

ME: 'But did you ask him at the end of treatment why he thought the treatment was not working?'

PSYCHOLOGIST: 'No, but I did not see the point at that stage.'

This conversation illustrates the arrogance of adherence to one model of care. The psychologist regarded herself as a successful therapist and, understandably, was getting peeved when the patient did not respond to her excellent care. But, however you looked at it, she had failed with her treatment and had not taken the trouble to find out the patient's views. 'Fail again, fail better', wrote Samuel Beckett, and if she had followed this dictum there might have been a better outcome.

Cause and pathology

It is possible to match the causes of mental disorder with levels in a similar way to that for treatment, but care is needed in defining cause or, to use its more technical synonym, aetiology. Just as an illness can show the features of all five levels at different times, in a similar way its cause can affect all five levels. A distinction is often made between 'causes' and 'triggering events' but this defines the level rather than a fundamental difference. Triggering events are usually at level one in the hierarchical model but they can lead to changes at other levels, and the nature of the disorder is the result of all these changes.

It is wrong to define any mental disorder by its apparent cause because of variability in response. Thus the term 'reactive depression' has been discarded because it implies a different type of depression than, for example, so-called 'endogenous depression'. If the 'reaction', whatever its nature, leads to significant deficiency in brain levels of certain amines (5-hydroxytryptamine and noradrenaline), then the clinical presentation will be the same as that for the (apparently) endogenously depressed patient. The reaction has taken place at level one but led to changes at level five, and these determine the nature of the depression.

Most mental disorders are reactive in one sense, in that their timing is determined by one or more external precipitants. It is underlying predisposition, or personality, that really decides the nature of the disorder and it is this level of aetiology that is associated with the presentation of illness (Tyrer, 2013a). Let us take an example to illustrate the importance of underlying predisposition in determining mental illness and how it is linked to aetiology.

Five people, whom we shall call A, B, C, D and E, are involved in a road traffic accident but not seriously injured. Subject A is of stable personality and has never had any mental illness. She recovers rapidly from the experience but for a short period prefers to travel by train rather than by car when she has a choice. Subject B is a somewhat insecure anxiety-prone man who has never adjusted to leaving his mother six years previously. He becomes much more anxious after the accident and has acute episodes of panic for no apparent reason. Subject C has a mother who has suffered from agoraphobia when she was a child. She has never had agoraphobia before but after the accident she developed some phobia of car travel. This later generalizes to all travelling outside the house so that she becomes severely agoraphobic. Subject D becomes depressed after the accident and cannot stop ruminating about death and his own mortality. Subject E has a father and grandfather who have had episodes of severe depression and he too has previously been in hospital with episodes of depression and hypomania. He appears not to react to the accident at first but a few weeks later he suddenly becomes overactive and restless, needing little sleep, shows elation and irritability alternately, and plans to build a spaceship to take him to Mars as the prospect of continued life on Earth is not exciting.

All these five people have been through the same experience but react differently because of different combinations of aetiological factors. Subject A reacts only to the accident, which can be said to be as much related to social forces as vehicular ones (level one). Subject B reactivates unresolved anxiety that stems from his relationship with his mother (level two). Subject C becomes agoraphobic with generalized avoidance, a pattern of behaviour she has developed at least as much from modelling herself on her agoraphobic mother as a child as on genetic predisposition (level three). Subject D develops persistent depressive thinking. Subject E enters a manic phase (level five) of his bipolar affective disorder for which the accident may be seen as an important, though non-specific, triggering event. But of course all five (level four) individuals have been through the same experience and so the aetio-logical factors of the first level are relevant to a varying degree in their resulting problems. Allowing room for simultaneous aetiological factors from different levels removes much controversy about the correct way to regard psychiatric illness. Although a condition may be triggered by social factors that is no reason to regard social forms of management as the only appropriate ones; it is the end result to the triggering that determines the best line of treatment.

Both types of pathology are similarly explained by using the hierarchy. Pathology does not only mean gross changes in bodily organs, such as the loss of brain cells and flattening of the grooves (sulci) in the brain in conditions such as senile dementia, it also describes abnormalities at other levels. So in psychoses well-known phrases such as 'ideas of reference' and 'delusional perception' are examples of descriptive psychopathology, and the maladaptive behaviour patterns of stage three, the dynamic psychopathology of stage two, and the social pathology of stage one are all manifestations of the form of illness. As long as one level of pathology is not applied to an inappropriate stage – for example, it would be nonsense to describe someone in a depressive stupor as displaying introjection and repression – then there is no difficulty in fitting pathology to the model.

Prevention

Prevention also follows the multi-model pattern of aetiology. It is appropriate for any preventive measure to be given provided that it matches the mental disorder at one level at least. Thus patients with recurrent episodes of mania and depression may take the treatment from stage five of our model, the drug lithium carbonate, even when they are completely well and outside the scope of our model altogether. But it would be inappropriate to give antidepressant tablets to a population living in squalid stressful conditions on the grounds that it would prevent them from becoming depressed. How do we go about using the hierarchical approach in practice? First of all there are some parts of each of the models described previously that can be incorporated into our model as general rules. The two aspects of the disease model that apply to all levels of illness are the need for a formalized assessment of every mental problem and the acceptance that in a doctor–patient relationship the patient has to adopt a sick role at some stage, even if it is only at the beginning.

The need for a formalized assessment will already be obvious to the reader. This assessment would be usually made at a first interview and involves a judicious mix of direct questions from the interviewer and spontaneous description of problems by the patient. A proper history of the problem and an assessment of the current mental state of the patient are essential parts, for without them much relevant material will remain undetected. The interviewer's assessment will be summarized in a formulation of the problem in aetiological, diagnostic and prognostic terms.

We should also like the doctor to describe which stage of the illness the patient has reached, as this will influence management; but as he will look in vain for any indication of this in psychiatric textbooks we shall have to ask him to use his own judgement in deciding this question. This judgement will require both an objective assessment of the patient's state and a recording of the patient's own views about his attitudes and feelings towards his problem. Sometimes these will vary: the patient may think his attacks of sweating and palpitations signify organic disease whereas the doctor will view them as anxiety symptoms. A sound knowledge of medicine and psychiatry is necessary to decide which interpretation is correct.

The acceptance of a sick role is implicit in every doctor–patient relationship. A person who seeks advice for health reasons (or for whom advice is sought by a third party) is at least temporarily in a dependent position. Something is recognized to be wrong and in need of putting right, and all workers in the caring professions, be they doctors, nurses, social workers, psychologists or occupational therapists, by offering any form of treatment are placing the patient in the sick role. Where the integrated model diverges from the disease model is in still giving responsibility to the patient for a substantial part of treatment. The patient is not merely a passive recipient of therapy but an active participant, to a lesser degree in stage five than stage one, but always having some active role.

The part of the psychodynamic model that applies throughout all phases of the hierarchical model is the awareness that the problems patients present to the doctor are only the tip of the iceberg. There are many unconscious, pre-conscious and conscious processes involved before the final form of the com-plaint is established, and this may be far removed from the underlying cause, as for example in the case of a hysterical symptom. Throughout assessment and treatment of a patient, the doctor has to be sensitive to other forms of communication and able to get across to the patient that he understands and is competent to deal with mental suffering. This quality is called empathy. The doctor also needs to be aware that the relationship he or she has with the patient can affect the outcome of therapy markedly, and by being sensitive to the nature of this relationship it can be used positively.

The cognitive-behavioural model reminds us that we too can determine our subsequent behaviour. 'Habit is the flywheel of society', wrote William James, and when habits are healthy all goes well. When they become mala-daptive they unfortunately tend to reinforce the maladaptation, and behav-ioural techniques are needed to modify them. Most of this does not pass under the form of specialized therapy. For example, the upbringing of almost all children involves reward for doing what is thought to be good and praise-worthy, and punishment for what is thought to be wrong. In some pathologi-cal states (e.g. pathological gambling) there is at times apparent punishment for good and reward for bad behaviour. Thinking can become disordered at the same time and the rational links between cognition and behaviour can be lost. The person with borderline personality disorder who has been rejected by her family and friends may only believe she has any status in society when she harms herself repeatedly ('at least other people take notice of me') and so her abnormal thinking and self-harming behaviour may be reinforced. A nudge towards more adaptive solutions is the task of the cognitive-behavioural model here.

The aspect of the social model that runs throughout the integrative model is the aetiological one. Many forms of psychiatric illness can be the result of social forces acting on vulnerable individuals. No patient can be studied in isolation and an awareness of social and cultural background is necessary to understand both the nature and form of psychiatric disorder. An increasingly important part of mental disorder is transcultural psychiatry, which recog-nizes that, although psychiatric illness may be fundamentally the same the world over, the relative frequency of disorder varies greatly from culture to culture, and the form that the illness takes even more so. Significantly altering social factors is difficult and again the needs of the individual have to be balanced against those of society. In major social reorganization such as planning a new town, the preventive importance of good planning in maintaining health deserves particular attention.

The task of matching the environment with the person is an essential component of nidotherapy, which derives directly from the social model. This approach could well be the philosophy of the social worker, as it is this discipline that his primary concern with balancing the needs of the individual with those of society. When these can be brought together through therapy then we have a valuable combination.

The doctor needs to incorporate all these points from our four previous models into the integrated hierarchical one. At initial assessment of the patient there will be concentration on getting enough information to summarize the problem formally. This will comprise factual, historical material derived from following the procedure given earlier in the account of the disease model (the data base) with corroboration of this, where necessary, from an independent informant, and an examination of the physical and mental state. The interview will also be used to build up a trusting relationship with the patient so that it does not consist of a series of brutal questions and answers but a gentle exploration of the problem. Even if the patient is apparently out of touch with his surroundings, whether or not he is suffering from a psychotic illness, the interview should proceed in the same gentle manner so that the foundations of mutual respect can be established. This may sound odd to those who have had to deal with violent people who are obviously 'mad' in the lay sense and psychotic in the medical one, but such patients can still appreciate good manners and careful handling although at the time they may not show it. The first interview usually sets the seal on the relationship at subsequent interviews and if it is handled badly the lost ground may never be recovered.

Once a diagnostic formulation and the level of illness has been established a plan of management is determined. This will depend on the nature and level of the illness and may consist of more than one approach for conditions that show elements of two levels. To a greater or lesser degree, depending on the state of the disorder, this plan will be discussed with the patient and approval sought. Approval may not always be given for conditions at level five of the model but the treatment may nevertheless have to be given compulsorily. In most instances approval for the passive component of treatment is readily given by the patient, for, after all, they make no contribution towards it. More difficulty may be reached in agreeing on the active component, and it may take some time before this is properly established. This does not prevent the passive form of treatment going ahead, but it should be discussed as soon as possible once a plan of management has been decided. It is fairly easy to treat a patient with a chronic drinking problem initially as the first stage is to withdraw the alcohol under supervision, but the patient's participation is so much more important in the later phases.

As treatment progresses the patient will pass down the hierarchy of the integrated model. There should be no difficulty in the therapist accommodating to this change in levels. He has already established the different levels of treatment with the patient and so does not give the impression of inconsistency or radical change of mind. The relationship between therapist and patient becomes more important in the cognitive-behavioural and psychodynamic stages of the model and is one reason for maintaining continuity of care in these stages. Major disruption can result if the patient is confronted by

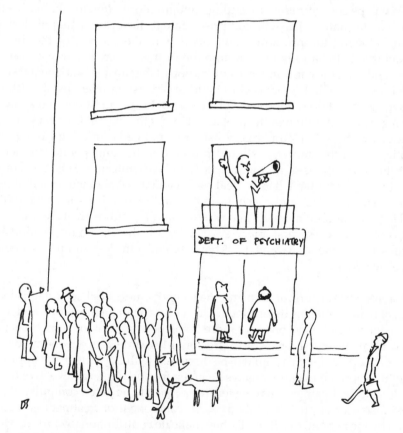

'It is not part of the professional's work to produce social reform . . . '

a different therapist at each succeeding level and establishing a relationship has to begin all over again. However, when the patient has reached the social level of illness some boundary would have to be drawn between the responsibility of mental health professionals and that of the wider community. It is not part of the professional's work to produce social reform, although many take up this issue independently of their mental health role. Psychiatrists in particular have sometimes overstretched their boundaries and incorporated their models into the whole framework of society. This is not wise.

Once the importance of looking at different stages of illness in different ways is appreciated, much of the bitter argument within the psychiatric profession and between other professionals disappears. The integrated approach does not mean a patient should be treated in the same way at all times, and dogmatic adherence to one particular model is a source of much conflict. Much depends on the training of professionals and who they see in their working lives. Social workers (apart from specialist mental health ones) see many of their clients at level one, psychoanalysts and psychotherapists treat their patients at level two, clinical psychologists practise their skills derived from the cognitive-behavioural model at levels three and four, and hospital-orientated psychiatrists see patients predominantly at the fifth level. This leads to a blinkered view of psychiatric existence. The social worker working in a rural team with drug misusers is often shocked when he or she hears of a client known for years to have major social difficulties is in a mental hospital and has been treated with ECT. This is an understandable response as the social worker's experience with the client has been almost entirely of the lower levels of the hierarchy. We all have the capacity to become psychotically ill and to require treatment at the disease level of the hierarchy. As one past president of the Royal College of Psychiatrists has put it, 'every citizen should have the right to be admitted against his or her will, to be treated without loss of dignity, in a first class psychiatric service' (Birley, 1991).

The patient with psychotic depression in hospital is very different from the one with problems at home seen by the social worker. Of course they are the same person, but the condition is as different from the ill person with pneumonia who is out of breath compared with his healthy self when he is breathless after running for a bus. If mental health professionals were able to see psychiatric patients at all levels of the model there would be much more understanding and less sniping at others' points of view.

All parts of the integrated model can link together harmoniously provided that it is clear which part is operative at any one time. This decision is not a fixed one, as advances in knowledge are always taking place that change our concepts of mental disorder. If, for example, it is confirmed that a certain patient with schizophrenia has permanent structural changes in the brain (an increasingly likely event from the latest research findings) (Chua and McKenna, 1995), it becomes much more appropriate to treat most of its manifestations according to stage five. The other four stages of the model still have a place once the major abnormality has been treated. There is also a major challenge for the model in the assessment and management of personality disorder. These conditions describe persistent maladaptive aspects of personality functioning that lead to impaired social function and influence the outcome of many mental illnesses. Personality disorder represents a challenge to the integrated model because it asks all parts of the model to work in unison. We are not pretending that the integrated model is going to solve all the difficulties of divergent schools in psychiatry, but we look on it as a good working hypothesis that should aid clinical practice. It should also give a theoretical base to the eclectic approach to psychiatry. The original eclectics were members of a school of Greek philosophy who had no doctrines of their own but borrowed ideas from other schools whenever it suited them. Not surprisingly they were not thought of very highly, and were considered to be third-rate philosophers who did not have sufficient originality to develop ideas of their own. The same image has tended to follow psychiatrists who regard themselves as eclectic. It may seem reasonable to choose the approach that best suits the situation, but if this is just a personal decision it lacks any general application and its practitioners are just dilettantes. We hope that the integrated model can be viewed as an eclectic's charter, giving a basis for good practice in psychiatry which can be developed and taught to others instead of accruing only from prolonged clinical experience.

CHILD AND COMMUNITY PSYCHIATRIC PRACTICE AS ONE MODEL FOR TEAMWORK

Although the practitioner can work in more than one way at a time, there are many reasons why the work is better shared. First, he or she may not be equally expert in everything that needs attention. Second, distributing work in a multidisciplinary way can be a more rational and economical way of bringing different sorts of skills to bear on the patient's case, and this is increasingly the philosophy behind community mental health teams being able to treat a large number of individuals. Third, it can be helpful to all concerned, professionals and the patient, to have more than one person's perspective, and in some complex cases someone able to stand back a little from the case. Fourth, there are times when two perfectly compatible approaches require two different sorts of therapist–patient relationship. For example, a young patient with severe obsessive-compulsive disorder may benefit from quite focused, structured, rather prescriptive behaviour therapy applied on an individual basis, and family therapy in which intra-family stresses, strains, anxieties and misunderstandings are explored in a less directive way.

To undertake these two approaches properly may well benefit from two people working together; indeed, some would say this would be essential.

The same would apply if, conversely, a patient with a personality disorder needed non-directive individual psychotherapy combined with quite firm and structured approaches such as mentalization-based treatment (Bateman and Fonagy, 2010), or dialectical behavior therapy (Linehan *et al.*, 2006).

Young people develop and undergo an extraordinary degree of change as they grow – physically, intellectually, in terms of the acquisition of skills and behaviour (e.g. reading, social skills) and in terms of what is expected of them. They also interact in complex ways first with their parents and later with wider aspects of their environment, e.g. with their friends and at school. Such changes of course affect the ways in which problems are expressed. To take only one obvious example, a 2-year-old baby will not toddle along to a doctor complaining of depression; a 17-year-old might; and a 12-year-old might or might not, and more likely would be taken by his or her parents, who may be more concerned about the child's symptoms than is the boy or girl. The nature of disorders in childhood and adolescence change too, so that what we think of as 'depression' might manifest as feeding problems in an infant, misbehaviour and school problems in middle childhood, and adult-type depressive symptoms in adolescence.

Thus things change as development proceeds: the child changes, the presentation of disorder changes, and quite probably at least some of the mechanisms underlying disorder change too. Childhood disorder is therefore conceptualized in developmental terms, rather than in the relatively stable concepts of adult psychiatry where changes in personality, disorder and circumstances can be less dramatic. Secondly, these changing internal and external influences and processes interact in a complicated way. Clarifying this requires information drawn from many different fields, including many different aspects of social, biological and psychological science; Rutter (1980) provides an excellent review of the field. In so far as the approach can be summed up in a sentence or two, it is based on the recognition that as development proceeds various inherent characteristics emerge and mature, and various external influences interact with these characteristics, which may then become modified.

However, these modified characteristics in turn influence other individual characteristics and the environment, and both of the latter may change too. This model, then, is one of a constant, complex interaction within the individual and between the individual and the external world. To take another example: a poor single woman, a heavy smoker, has her child in a poor neighbourhood where obstetric and paediatric facilities are less than ideal.

Her low self-esteem and general level of expectations means that she does not use the reasonable antenatal advice and care that is available, and she does not complain about poor service from doctors and nurses. Her own family background has taught her to be compliant. The baby is born somewhat underweight and rather hard to manage: he has feeding problems and is easily upset and is slow to develop predictable habits. The vulnerable mother loses heart and gets irritable with the child, which makes matters worse for both. They upset each other, and in the next few years she is more or less constantly depressed and the child is irritable, enuretic and overactive, the problems for which he is referred. He goes to a rough school in a rough neighbourhood, learns little and goes from bad to worse.

The 'advice' implied by this sketch, whether as health advice and education, as social policy, or as care in the individual case, clearly includes matters to do with basic physical health and care for mothers and babies, the upbringing of children, the psychology of motherhood and the quality and accessibility of obstetric and paediatric services; and matters to do with schooling. In addition, the child may or may not have a clinical disorder.

These complexities are organized in diagnostic assessment by using the multiaxial approach described earlier, in which factors are teased out in terms of individual disorder, if any, developmental delay, intellectual level, physical health and psychosocial circumstances. The formulation in child and adolescent psychiatry is made in similar terms. Earlier, we described the process of assessment as consisting partly of description of the problem in ordinary language, and partly of explanation in which complex models are used. If we take this approach we will often be left with two sets of problems – problems which, once clarified, can be dealt with by (for example) a referred child's parents and teachers; and problems for which psychiatric help is more appropriate. This is where teamwork comes in and where an integrated model of care is useful. All psychiatrists, not just those in child and adolescent psychiatry, have to work with a range of other professionals, those from inside and outside the mental health services, to meet the needs of referred patients. Team-working characteristically involves joint assessment and allocation so that a key worker from an appropriate discipline takes on the main clinical responsibility. For example, if the child in the above example was referred to a psychiatrist, it could well turn out that the psychiatrist, an educational psychologist, schoolteachers and the local practice's health visitor would need to collaborate with each other and with the child and family to help school and parents handle the child along sensible and consistent lines. In a case like this the psychiatrist may not need to do any clinical work with the referred child, but simply take an advisory or consultative role, perhaps with health visitor and school. Alternatively, he might work directly with the child, the mother, or both together – in which case he would be doing family work. This may consist of family therapy, using a systems-based or psychodynamic model; or he may help the mother using a behavioural or cognitive approach (Steinberg, 1983, 1986). Steinberg, arguing that modern medicine is not only complex but becoming increasingly so, has suggested that the multidimensional, consultative approach taken routinely in child psychiatry (Steinberg, 2005) could be a useful model to include in general medical training (Steinberg, 2004), although this may be a somewhat idiosyncratic position.

The concept of case or care management enshrines this notion of team-working with appropriate levels of responsibility. Good team-working requires the integrated model we have put forward if it is not to lead to sterile arguments between disciplines that serve only to fragment care. There are many ways of organizing good team-working and case management (Onyett, 1992), and it is important to recognize that it is not necessarily easy or straightforward (Parry-Jones, 1986; Steinberg, 1986).

COMPLEXITY IN MEDICINE AND PSYCHIATRY

It is often both necessary and interesting in psychiatry to 'reframe' a problem, in other words to shift the goalposts – for example, focusing for a time on anxiety, indecisiveness and conflict in a patient's family and their direct consequences on a patient's progress (if only in whether or not he takes his medication reliably), rather than as a kind of peripheral issue. Medicine as a whole, and not least psychiatry, has recently been subjected to this kind of scrutiny or, if you like the philosophical term, deconstruction. Thus although doctors and other health workers, patients, administrators and politicians tend to blame each other for the shortcomings and general turbulence of modern health services, the real problem is that the whole issue of health and treatment is immensely complex and constantly verging on the chaotic.

'Chaos' and 'complexity' in this context mean rather different things to what might be supposed; it does not mean a complete shambles, indeed compared with chaos and complexity a shambles might seem rather neat and tidy. *Complexity* represents a relatively recent way of conceptualizing how living systems function: they are multifactorial, the many factors interact with each other and with the environment, the interactions are non-linear (see below), and as a result of this complex interaction new properties of the systems emerge (= 'emergent behaviours') which cannot be explained by examination of any single element in the system (Burton, 2002). They are also open systems, that is to say *the observer becomes part of the system*, a notion which is unsettling for the nineteenth-century philosophy of science on which much of modern psychiatry is based, though as it happens is taken for granted in psychoanalytic theory, family therapy and quantum physics.

Complex systems can adapt to their environment, which is how they have evolved, but can readily become chaotic, typically, for example, when something new is added (e.g. an excess of alcohol). They then cease to adapt and change unpredictably and – the essence of chaos – beyond measurement by the kinds of calculations we can do. Floods, crowds and traffic may behave chaotically in equivalent ways. There is a growing literature on complexity and chaos, and Gleick (1987) provides a good introduction.

The notion of *non-linearity* is the key to understanding complexity and chaos. Much of what we are taught in medicine and psychiatry is that A causes B, which is then recognized by symptoms C as diagnosis D, and hence the point of treatment E. This model of understanding remains as important for much of clinical work as, say, Newtonian and nineteenth-century physics provides the right conceptual models for building a bridge. However, just as nuclear physics needs the more complex and chaotic models of quantum physics, modern medical care benefits from a different kind of model entirely – the *general systems model* in which, at its simplest, A causes B, C and D, and C and D in turn affect not only A, hence full circle, but Dr X the clinician too.

The patient's relatives may be behaving in ways which encourage the clinician to keep changing the drugs rather than looking at ways in which the relatives might change. One might reasonably comment that a busy psychiatrist might not have (a) the time to go into all that, nor (b) the inclination or interest, nor (c) the training; it might even clash with the team's or the institution's ethos. However, far from representing side-issues, these are key elements E, F, G, H and I too in our elaborately reciprocating system, which shows how complex health services can be.

Methicillin-resistant *Staphylococcus aureus* (MRSA) infection in hospitals is a good case to analyse (or deconstruct) using complex models. The linear model (diagnose and prescribe) is insufficient, and instead we have to consider issues like attitudes, education, behaviour (moving patients from unit to unit, visiting times, what to wear in the ward, sitting on the bed) and job descriptions and contracts (e.g. of ward sister and cleaning services) as well as hoping that pharmacology will come up with something.

All of which may seem daunting, but science and medicine were never easy.

CONSULTATIVE APPROACHES TO COMPLEXITY

The problem with the word 'consultation' is that it can mean just about any conversation or interview with anybody. For the purposes of this book we would like to identify two kinds of consultation, the traditional *clinical consultation*, usually based for good time-honoured and pragmatic reasons on the linear model ('what seems to be the trouble?'), and the more recently developed kind of consultation variously known as mental health consultation (Caplan, 1970) or organizational consultation (e.g. Cooklin, 1999), or 'inter-professional consultation' or consultative work (Steinberg, 1993, 2000a, 2005), a variety of terminology itself indicative of the range and complexity which this kind of consultation tries to encompass.

A reasonable technical term to be getting on with may be *systems consultation*, as the task is to explore the kinds of complex, non-linear and sometimes chaotic systems outlined above. It was developed not as a clinical tool (indeed it is the antithesis of the clinical model) but as a way of looking beyond the clinical and into other significant areas. It may be described as a method of joint enquiry (typically between two or more healthcare workers) into the wider ramifications of a problem; for example, a child psychiatrist consulting with a teacher and a psychologist about a child's intractable misbehaviour in school may discover not attention-deficit hyperkinetic disorder, but problems concerning how the child is taught, in the parenting style at home and family relationships generally, in parent–school relationships, and in the child's relationships with his peers. These kinds of findings (by no means uncommon in psychiatry) may or may not necessarily replace the clinical diagnosis, but can augment it and provide additional worthwhile lines of management, some of which (e.g. encouraging parent–school collaboration and consistency) may enable a clinical treatment to begin to work. Thus the consultative process can both discover non-clinical ways of helping and act as a complement to clinical approaches.

This kind of inter-professional collaboration, which may be defined as a joint enquiry into what is wanted, what is needed (which may be rather different) and what is possible (different again), can provide an effective and productive way into the shadowy jungle of complex healthcare systems (Steinberg, 2005). It is a strategy for developing problem-clarifying and problem-solving techniques across disciplines, rather than relying on each discipline's own preferred conceptual models; and indeed the special language of consultative work, its lingua franca, should be plain English (or whatever the demotic language happens to be). This can be the biggest challenge of all.

The advantages of the consultative approach described here are that it acknowledges a wider range of possibly influential factors having a bearing on the case, and strategies to handle them; that the user of the consultation service (the consultee) remains as far as possible in charge of the 'case' and continues using his or her own experience and skills; thus the child in the above example might well become better handled at home and at school rather than having to become a patient; moreover, another referral or 'move' is avoided (there might be no need to see the psychiatrist at all); and the whole process is a teaching exercise for consultant and consultee, both ending up knowing more for the next time about similar cases. On the one hand, being relatively new, this model of working may seem a cumbersome alternative to clinical work; however, it is a way of rationalizing the use of clinical skills, clinic time and of course waiting lists, especially as in psychiatry, where diagnoses and specific needs are not clear-cut, and as its founder Caplan (1970) suggested, it has a preventive function too. As a means of systematic enquiry into everything possibly bearing on a case it is also a powerful tool for teaching and enquiry.

Approaches along consultative lines may prove to have a place in recent moves towards 'patient empowerment' (Coulter, 2003; Spiers, 2003) which is by no means as straightforward a development as it seems. It can sometimes have the opposite effect to that intended, for example when perceived by patients as being yet another idea controlled by and within the patronage of doctors (e.g. Salmond and Hall, 2004). It might be that the consultative model, developed though it was as a peer–peer exercise for professional workers, could be transposed to the clinician–patient relationship, and provide a workable and adaptive model for negotiating patient autonomy. The consultative model would be in a strong position to make the most of the clinician's expertise and experience *and* that of the patient (by negotiating what A and B can contribute) without diminishing the authority of either, without prior assumptions about the balance of the outcome, and in clarifying the crucial issue of informed consent (Steinberg, 1992, 2000b, 2005).

PATIENTS' VIEWS AND MODELS

We do not know how many patients currently or recently treated or involved in using mental health services may read this book, but we are expecting at least some to do so. After all, it is difficult to avoid one of the labels of mental illness being attached to us at some time in our lives, however hard we try to brush it off and pretend it is not there. We have tried to cover this possibility by explaining in relatively straightforward language the ways in which mental health professionals think about their craft and how best to use it to maximum effect. We are not sure that we have, as to write comprehensively yet without jargon is remarkably difficult. Nevertheless, this section is an attempt to widen the picture by approaching models from the patients' viewpoint.

A psychiatric patient is now a consumer in business terms, although this is usually an aspiration rather than a fact. If he or she does not like what is on offer there is the option, at least in theory, of going elsewhere to get a better deal. This certainly happens in private practice, and is becoming more common even in the public arena. Ideally we would like to be able to help to match the expectations of the patient by getting a practitioner who would employ the appropriate model of care to complete the match. But we have to be aware of the different ways in which patients come into contact with psychiatric services and have to recognize that choice is not always available, at least not at first. Let us look at some typical scenarios.

The compulsory admission

For the patient admitted as an emergency under a compulsory order there appears to be little choice in care. But there is more than you might think. Firstly, some patients choose the time of admission under an order even though it appears to be an emergency. 'I realized that things were getting impossible with my paranoia so I just took all my clothes off – it's the only way you can get the attention of the police in Paddington,' said one of our patients as she was recovering from her psychotic illness, frankly admitting that she had generated the crisis. And she was right. Down the road from her address at almost the same time the humorist Spike Milligan, no stranger to mental illness himself, was confirming her hypothesis in verse:

> 'He danced with a monkey
> He danced with a cat
> And he danced with a man
> In a big black hat
> He danced with a Muslim
> He danced with a Jew
> And he danced with a Chinaman
> Six foot two
> Then he took all his clothes off
> And he danced all day
> That's when they came
> And took him away.'
>
> (Milligan, 2004; verse written in 1994)

Our patient also realized very quickly that if she 'behaved herself' in hospital and agreed with everything offered that an early discharge might follow. It did indeed, but unfortunately she had recurrent brief psychotic episodes and really wanted to endure them in a sympathetic environment without the need to come into hospital or to be treated according to the disease model. 'You have a psychosis; there is no successful treatment for this apart from antipsychotic drugs, so you must have antipsychotic drugs,' was the constant refrain when she asked for an alternative approach. So she adopted a different tack. She persuaded a psychiatrist (PT) to let her stay under care without taking drugs and in the knowledge that almost certainly she would have further episodes, but if she was in the right sort of supportive environment (now part of the nidotherapy approach) she would be able to 'ride them' at home until she improved. She made an excellent case for this approach and has hardly had a day in hospital since (Tyrer, 2000); this is one of the few occasions when the social model has trumped the disease one.

The resistant problem

In this scenario the patient can choose the timing of the therapeutic approach much more confidently, but there is difficulty in choosing the right person (or team) to give the treatment. It is here where a reasonable knowledge of the models discussed in this book will be of great potential help. The sufferer from any mental disorder has a great deal to overcome in understanding the best way to deal with their condition, but they often feel instinctively that certain approaches are right and others are wrong. Despite this, the wrong decisions are often made.

Why Virginia Woolf, the celebrated novelist, and her family (who published all the early texts on psychoanalysis) should have chosen Dr George Savage, former physician superintendent of the Bethlem Hospital, a worthy manager but a limited physician, to treat her recurrent depression rather than one of the many psychoanalysts well known to her family (Virginia even met Sigmund Freud when he came to London after leaving Austria) is difficult to comprehend. Dr Savage's advice was the subject of scorn and ridicule to Virginia, indicated by his proxy description in the form of Sir William Bradshaw (a private Harley Street psychiatrist) in her novel, *Mrs Dalloway*, who advises a soldier, Septimus Smith, with likely post-traumatic stress to be admitted to hospital compulsorily after a 45-minute consultation as he has 'a complete physical and mental breakdown' and treatment 'is merely a question of rest, of rest, rest, rest; a long rest in bed' (Woolf, 1925). To avoid admission Septimus jumps out of the window and kills himself. Virginia herself was always being advised by Dr Savage to have long rests away from the stresses of London, and frequently retired to her retreat in Richmond, but eventually responded in the same way as Septimus. Poor Dr Savage was even got at by his public patients when he was at the Bethlem Hospital. A Mr William Budd, a manic-depressive (now bipolar) patient, one of the early pioneers of the user movement in psychiatry, wrote to him from his hospital bed in 1886:

> 'Dear Doctor, when the trumpet sounds
> And God proclaims the judgement day
> You'll try I know to be at least
> Some fifty miles or more away
> 'Twill be no use, no tree no bush

Will hide from God's searching eye
With other Savages you'll have
To toddle up your luck to try.'

(Gale and Howard, 2003, p. 22)

So, if you are the patient wanting to get the best of deals from the service, please ensure the right match. Get as much information you can about the potential therapists available, do whatever you can to test out which models are likely to be most productive with your disorder, and set out your stall. Challenge the doctor when you feel it is justified, and make sure the multi-disciplinary team are fully on board. A good team, as should be clear from the description above, will contain different opinions and these will be expressed openly – the ability to show open dissent is what distinguishes a proper multidisciplinary team from one that is merely a multi-agency one – and so, if you feel you are not getting your point over successfully, you can persuade others in the team to take up your cause.

Self-help

For those with less serious but nonetheless chronically handicapping condi-tions, self-help may be the answer. This is not only suitable for those with an aversion to external help from a live therapist, but also for those who wish to stay in control of their treatment and want to proceed at a pace of their choos-ing. The best-known book of self-help for the common mental disorders, *Self Help for Your Nerves* (1995), by Claire Weekes. has helped millions (yes, mil-lions) of people without any other need for mental health input. There is now a host of self-help materials that can be of great help – provided you know where to look. There are now many ways of finding the right self-help mate-rials. If you are clear about the name of the disorder you are suffering from it is relatively easy to find out the name of self-help organizations (most will be registered charities) that are relevant to you. Other general websites (e.g. Psych Web) may also be accessed. The relevant sites, and recommended books, should give the clue to the models that you feel are most appropriate for your condition. In the United Kingdom, there is an excellent organiza-tion, the National Institute for Health and Care Excellence (NICE) (www. nice.org.uk), that gives unbiased advice based on the most up-to-date infor-mation on treatments for all of the important mental disorders, ranging from drug treatment, to psychotherapy, to cognitive-behavioural therapy (which can be given in book and computer format without the need for a therapist) (Wright and Wright, 1997; Williams and Garland, 2002; Proudfoot *et al.*, 2003), to general management, with recommended good practice for each of them. However, recommended good practice is only a guide. As you will gather from the variation illustrated in this book, treatments for ailments are like horses for courses, and one may be anathema to one but helpful to another.

MODELS OF CARE

One of the lessons that has been learnt somewhat painfully during the development of multidisciplinary work is that successful integration of methods and models requires a careful balance between shared basic knowledge and philosophy on the one hand and genuinely different skills and roles on the other. If everyone in the team thinks exactly alike then the team, its clientele and its trainees do not really have the benefit of a multidisciplinary perspective. The strength of multidisciplinary work lies in the coordination and successful application of a diverse range of skills and experience.

The management and leadership of such teams is beyond this book's brief, but it is important to recognize some of the quite different models of care involved, not least because failure to recognize that they are different can lead to confused role-blurring and muddle. Out-patient or sessional care implies that something can be 'carried', so to speak, by the patient from one appointment to the next, be it the maintenance of medication, the practising of behavioural approaches, or the internal psychological work done between psychotherapeutic sessions. Family work is also usually sessional, but here the problem and ways of handling it are shared, and not just left to the individual. Home-based care can be an extension of individual or family work, and follows when for whatever reason of organization or efficiency it appears to make more sense for the therapist or team to see how things are being handled in real home life and to adapt treatment accordingly. This has particular advantages for some groups who are, to put it at its most polite, not particularly good at keeping in touch with services by the usual

---

MODELS FOR CARE: WHERE CARE HAPPENS

- In the home
- Out-patient, general practice and clinic care
- Day care
- Residential care – supervision of, assistance with and training in ordinary living skills
- Residential care: the therapeutic community – supervision of, assistance with and training in inter-personal and emotional self-management
- Residential care: the hospital – availability of clinical skills for assessment, observation and treatment; the implication is that the observations and management needed require specifically clinical skills, e.g. medical and nursing, and laboratory support. This does not necessarily indicate severity of illness, because round-the-clock attention may be needed in particular circumstances for observation, for trials of treatment under safe conditions or for sustaining behaviour therapy

channels, and who usually have recurrent severe mental illness and poor engagement with services (Burns and Firn, 2002).

Residential care implies sufficient severity of illness or disability to justify supportive and appropriately trained care staff on the spot, providing supervised and assisted living.

MODELS OF PROFESSIONAL WORK

It would invite greater controversy than a slim volume can prepare itself against to attempt to define, even in broad terms, what the role of the psychiatrist should be compared with, say, that of psychologists, community physicians, nurses and the many other professionals engaged in the psychiatric field. One of us once prepared for a lecture a slide listing no fewer than 17 fields of psychosocial work, and found of course that he had still left out the jobs of a substantial number of his protesting audience.

Perhaps one useful distinction is between those who tend to work sessionally and by timetable or appointment with individuals or groups, and those whose task is more to do with maintaining a helpful environment, for example in the home, in residential care or in a hospital. We have already suggested some basic differences between supervised and supported living, for example in a home for the elderly, and the sort of reasons that justify hospital care. An intermediate type of setting of particular relevance to psychiatry is where the environment as a whole is maintained as one in which people in difficulties can learn and develop. Thus, over the years, therapeutic communities have developed in which workers from fields such as psychiatry, psychology, nursing and social work have staffed and led settings where group expectations, group example and, when needed, group pressure are engineered to help the residents with their emotional states, behaviour and self-management.

The archetypal sessional worker was the doctor, coming and going to clinics and ward rounds once a week or so. Similarly, the tradition of nursing grew out of the need in hospitals for staff to look after, feed and clean sick people round the clock and make sure that medicines were taken and dressings changed. The nursing role has developed enormously since the early days, and now extends both into sessional therapeutic care in hospitals, clinics and the home, and into shaping up residential care into the particular type of overall therapeutic environment needed by different patient groups. Thus psychiatric nurses are increasingly experienced in group and organizational skills as well as in the more traditional models of treatment, and may enter further training in behaviour therapy, social skills training, family therapy and the individual psychotherapies.

What is now very clear, and it is a positive development since the first edition of this book in 1987, is that the idiosyncratic practitioner who is out of step with colleagues and whose practice is dogmatic and bizarre now has no place to hide in a developed mental health service; and yet at the same time as service must allow for individuality and innovation, and there is some evidence that now that mental health services, after developing quickly and proactively in their first years of innovation, and now become too rigid (Tyrer, 2013b). The inappropriate use of a single model of mental illness is now almost part of the history of the subject. We are all working much better together in practice.

CONCLUSION

The reader who has persevered to the end of this book will now understand why we still have to have models in psychiatry. The single model outlined here is a complex one, which requires understanding of all the other models and so it is unlikely to be popular when we have simple ones that can be

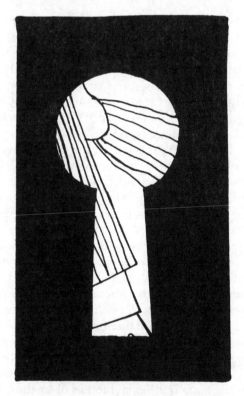

'. . . those who imprison themselves within the confines of one model only have the perspective of the keyhole . . .'

taken off the shelf and developed for specific purposes. We are living in a specialist's world and every patient wants to see an expert in the field of his or her illness. This may be possible for physical disease but it is far too complicated for mental disorder and every patient needs to be reminded that they are really in the driving seat when it comes to deciding what approach should be made in an individual case. And patients do not align themselves to simple models; they revel in the complexity that makes each one of their problems unique. So remember, we may be proud to be specialists, but our patients remain generalists, and are ever likely to stay so.

Our advice to the serious student, practitioner and patient is to retain an open mind about the helpfulness in clinical practice of the different models, and not to be seduced by the superficial attractiveness of one, however well presented. Diversity is the stuff of psychiatry, and those who imprison themselves within the confines of one model only have the perspective of the keyhole, a perspective that is stimulating at first but which without the wider view is seriously limiting. Good models are vehicles for progress, not icons to be worshipped, and we must never allow them to become our masters.

REFERENCES

American Psychiatric Association (1994) *Diagnostic and Statistical Manual for Mental Disorders*, 4th revision. American Psychiatric Association, Washington, DC.

Bateman, A. and Fonagy, P. (2010) Mentalization based treatment for borderline personality disorder. *World Psychiatry*, **9**, 11–15.

Birley, J.L.T. (1991) Psychiatrists and citizens. *British Journal of Psychiatry*, **159**, 1–6.

Blashfield, R.K. and Fuller, A.K. (1996) Predicting the DSM-V. *Journal of Nervous and Mental Diseases*, **184**, 4–7.

Burns, T. and Firn, M. (2002) *Assertive Outreach in Mental Health: A Manual for Practitioners*. Oxford University Press, Oxford.

Burns, T., Yeeles, K., Molodynski, A., et al. (2011) Pressures to adhere to treatment ('leverage') in English mental healthcare. *British Journal of Psychiatry*, **199**, 145–50.

Burton, C. (2002) Introduction to complexity. In: K. Sweeney and F. Griffiths (eds) *Complexity and Healthcare: An Introduction*. Radlciffe Publishing, Abingdon.

Caplan, G. (1970) *The Principles and Practice of Mental Health Consultation*. Tavistock, London.

Chua, S.E. and McKenna, P.J. (1995) Schizophrenia – a brain disease? A critical review of structural and functional cerebral abnormality in the disorder. *British Journal of Psychiatry*, **166**, 563–582.

Cooklin, A. (ed.) (1999) *Changing Organisations: Clinicians as Agents of Change*. Karnac Books, London.

Cooper, J.E., Kendall, R.E., Gurland, B.J., Sharpe, L., Copeland, J.R.M., Simon, R. (1972) *Psychiatric Diagnosis in New York and London: A Comparative Study of Mental Hospital Admissions*. Maudsley Monograph 20. Oxford University Press, Oxford.

Coulter, A. (2003) Patients, power and responsibility. Review of Spiers, J. (2003) *Journal of the Royal Society of Medicine*, **96**, 512–513.

Craddock, N. and Owen, M.J. (2005) The beginning of the end for the Kraepelinian dichotomy. *British Journal of Psychiatry*, **186**, 364–366.

Foucault, M. (1967) *Madness and Civilisation*. Tavistock, London.

Gale, C. and Howard, R. (2003) *Presumed Curable: An Illustrated Casebook of Victorian Psychiatric Patients in Bethlem Hospital*. Wrightson Biomedical Publishing, Petersfield.

Gleick, J. (1987) *Chaos: Making a New Science*. Sphere Books, Penguin, London.

Lewis, A. (1953) Health as a social concept. *British Journal of Sociology*, **4**, 109–124.

Linehan, M.M., Comtois, K.A., Murray, A.M., *et al.* (2006) Two-year randomized controlled trial and follow-up of dialectical behavior therapy vs therapy by experts for suicidal behaviors and borderline personality disorder. *Archives of General Psychiatry*, **63**, 757–766.

Mulder, C.L., Uitenbroek, D., Broer, J., *et al.* (2008) Changing patterns in emergency involuntary admissions in the Netherlands in the period 2000–2004. *International Journal of Law and Psychiatry*, **31**, 331–336.

Onyett, S. (1992) *Case Management in Mental Health*. Chapman and Hall, London.

Parry-Jones, W. (1986) Multi-disciplinary work: help or hindrance? In: D. Steinberg (ed.) *The Adolescent Unit: Work and Teamwork in Adolescent Psychiatry*. Wiley, Chichester.

Milligan, S. (2004) In: N. Farnes (ed.) *The Compulsive Spike Milligan*, p.394. Fourth Estate, London.

Proudfoot, J., Goldberg, D., Mann, A., Everitt, B., Marks, I. and Gray, J.A. (2003) Computerized, interactive, multimedia cognitive-behavioural program for anxiety and depression in general practice. *Psychological Medicine*, **33**, 217–227.

Ramon, S. (1985) *Psychiatry in Britain: Meaning and Policy*. Croom Helm, London.

Rutter, M. (ed.) (1980) *Developmental Psychiatry*. Heinemann, London.

Salkovskis, P.M. (2002) Empirically grounded clinical interventions: cognitive-behavioural therapy progresses through a multi-dimensional approach to clinical science. *Behavioural and Cognitive Psychotherapy*, **30**, 3–9.

Salmond, P. and Hall, G. (2004) Patient empowerment or the emperor's new clothes? *Journal of the Royal Society of Medicine*, **97**, 53–56.

Spiers, J. (2003) *Patients, Power and Responsibility: The First Principles of Consumer-driven Reform*. Radcliffe Publishing, Abingdon.

Spiegel, A. (2005) The dictionary of disorder: how one man revolutionized psychiatry. *New Yorker*, January 3.

Steinberg, D. (1983) *The Clinical Psychiatry of Adolescence: Clinical Work from a Social and Developmental Perspective*. Wiley, Chichester.

Steinberg, D. (ed.) (1986) *The Adolescent Unit: Work and Teamwork in Adolescent Psychiatry*. Wiley, Chichester.

Steinberg, D. (1989) *Interprofessional Consultation*. Blackwell Scientific, Oxford.

Steinberg, D. (1992) Informed consent: consultation as a basis for collaboration between disciplines and between professions and their patients. *Journal of Interprofessional Care*, **61**, 43–48.

Steinberg, D. (1993) Consultative work in child and adolescent psychiatry. In: M.E. Garralda (ed.) *Managing Children with Psychiatric Problems*. BMJ Publishing, London.

Steinberg, D. (2000a) The child psychiatrist as consultant to schools and colleges. In: M. Gelder, J. Lopez-Ibor and H. Andreasen (eds) *New Oxford Textbook of Psychiatry*. Oxford University Press, Oxford.

Steinberg, D. (2000b) *Letters from the Clinic. Letter Writing in Clinical Practice for Mental Health Professionals*. Brunner-Routledge, London.

Steinberg, D. (2004) Child and adolescent psychiatry – a model for medical teaching. *Journal of the Royal Society of Medicine*, **97**, 545–546.

Steinberg, D. (2005) *Complexity and Healthcare and the Language of Consultation: Exploring the Other Side of Medicine*. Radcliffe Publishing, Abingdon.

Szasz, T.S. (1961) *The Myth of Mental Illness*. Harper and Row, New York.

Tyrer, P. (2000) Patients who have changed my practice: the case for patient-based evidence versus evidence-based medicine. *International Journal of Psychiatry in Clinical Practice*, **4**, 253–255.

Tyrer, P. (2012) DSM – 100 words. *British Journal of Psychiatry*, **200**, 67.

Tyrer, P., Mitchard, S., Methuen, C. and Ranger, M. (2003) Treatment-rejecting and treatment-seeking personality disorders: Type R and Type S. *Journal of Personality Disorders*, **17**, 265–270.

Tyrer, P. (2013a) Personality dysfunction is the cause of recurrent non-cognitive mental disorder: a testable hypothesis. *Personality and Mental Health* (in press).

Tyrer, P. (2013b) A solution to the ossification of community psychiatry. *The Psychiatrist* (in press).

Weekes, C. (1995) *Self Help for Your Nerves*. Thorsons, London.

Williams, C.J. and Garland, A. (2002) A cognitive behaviour therapy assessment model for use in everyday clinical practice. *Advances in Psychiatric Treatment*, **8**, 172–179.

Woolf, V. (1925) *Mrs Dalloway*. Hogarth Press, London.

World Health Organization (1992) *International Classification of Diseases*, 10th edn. WHO, Geneva.

Wright, J.H. and Wright, A.S. (1997) Computer-assisted psychotherapy. *Journal of Psychotherapy Practice and Research*, **6**, 315–329.

APPENDIX: TEACHING EXERCISE

In teaching the different models we often use examples derived from clinical practice condensed into case vignettes. Commonly we divide students into four groups, each of which is given one of the models to apply to each example. After joint discussion, each group decides on the application of their model to the problem and a spokesperson is elected to debate that model subsequently. Here is one of the examples and a summary of the approaches followed by each model. Of course there are many other similar examples illustrated in the rest of this book. The students should be instructed to look at this as a dramatic exercise in which each is trying to persuade other groups that their model is the best, so a good adversarial debate is ideal.

Clinical example

A man aged 24 presents to a psychiatric clinic complaining that he is being persecuted. His family have been continually criticizing him because he only has a clerical job and they wanted him to become a doctor. He now feels that they are talking to him even when he is on his own. They make derogatory comments such as 'He's going into the office to waste time all day filling in forms. Why doesn't he do something useful for once?' He believes that they may have set up a computer-linked surveillance system to keep him under constant observation and can imagine a line from George Orwell's *1984* being repeated over and over: 'Big brother is watching you.' Because of this interference he cannot concentrate and is thinking of giving up his job.

Models for Mental Disorder: Conceptual Models in Psychiatry, Fifth Edition. Peter Tyrer.
© 2013 John Wiley & Sons, Ltd. Published 2013 by John Wiley & Sons, Ltd.

Interpretation – disease model

He has paranoid schizophrenia with classical delusions about being watched and persecuted and also has auditory hallucinations in the third person, one of the core (first-rank) symptoms of schizophrenia. There is no doubt that he has a serious disease and needs treatment with antipsychotic drugs to correct his abnormal dopamine metabolism. These will suppress his schizophrenic symptoms and return him to a normal state.

Interpretation – psychodynamic model

This man has never grown up and is arrested at an infantile stage of development. He continues to be regarded as a young child by his overbearing, controlling mother and father and they continue to dominate his life. Everything he has done has been designed to please them and, even though he has now grown up and left home, this control persists. He needs psychodynamic psychotherapy to explore his real feelings and wishes and decide on his own identity in a hostile world.

Interpretation – cognitive-behavioural model

This man is behaving as though he has schizophrenia but his behaviour is maladaptive and unhelpful and he is misinterpreting his thoughts. He naturally feels upset about the antagonism his parents are showing towards him but he is exaggerating their influence on him. He needs to be reminded of the positive things about his life – his job, his friends, his hobbies. Do other people apart from his family think he is useless? Would his boss continue to employ him if he was no good? By building up a positive framework of thinking the negative impact of his family can be nullified. Getting more success in his chosen work will improve his self-confidence and aid this approach.

Interpretation – social model

Society, mainly in the form of this man's family, has created this apparent illness. He has been brought up by his snobbish parents to believe that only professional jobs are worthwhile and all others are demeaning. His own abilities and needs have been ignored and the special niche that he could develop for himself in society has never been explored properly. He needs to be removed from his family and helped to realize that he is no worse and no better than other human beings, and given a chance to blossom.

Afterwards, the group as a whole could discuss how an integrated model would be preferable in the treatment of this person.

GLOSSARY OF TERMS

Adjustment disorder: These are conditions which occur in response to an external stressor and which would not have occurred if the stressor had not been present. The term is not often used in mental illness services but these conditions are important as they usually do not need specific treatment as they will resolve spontaneously or with very little additional assistance.

Agoraphobia: This literally means fear of public places (often falsely translated as fear of open spaces). It was originated by the German psychiatrist, Carl Westphal, in 1871, and is derived from the Greek 'agora' (market-place) and phobia. This was an apt description as market-places can be very busy and constricting (inability to escape (claustrophobia) is one of the agoraphobic's fears) and also threateningly empty. Agoraphobia normally includes fears of travelling by public transport, crossing major roads, going out of the house and visiting shops and supermarkets.

Anomie: The state described by Durkheim as the relative absence of clear social and moral norms in those who are in this state. Said by Durkheim to be particularly absent at times of isolation and in those who are suicidal. Part of the aim of care using the social model is to remove anomie by promoting mutual interdependence between an individual and his or her close and wider social network so that protective bonds are developed.

Archetypes: A term from Jungian psychology meaning the inherited psychoneurological *predisposition* to form particular images and items. It does not mean directly inherited images and ideas. Such innate ideas and images tend to organize experience in innately predetermined patterns.

Behaviour therapy: The description of planned alteration in behaviour using approaches derived from learning theory whereby maladaptive behaviour is changed to more appropriate adaptive forms.

Behaviour activation therapy: A simple expansion of the behavioural aspect of cognitive therapy that has been particularly adapted for depression.

Models for Mental Disorder: Conceptual Models in Psychiatry, Fifth Edition. Peter Tyrer.
© 2013 John Wiley & Sons, Ltd. Published 2013 by John Wiley & Sons, Ltd.

Behaviourism: The term introduced by John B. Watson to describe the scientific study of behaviour as an important part of psychological science.

Bipolar affective disorder: A serious mental illness (formerly called manic-depressive psychosis) in which there are clear episodes of elevated mood (mania or hypomania (a lesser degree of mania)) or lowered mood (depression) with normal function in between.

Collective unconscious: The Jungian notion that at a certain very fundamental level the human race shares archetypes (q.v.) because they are universal products of the same kinds of brain.

Complexes: Collections of interacting conscious and unconscious feelings and ideas which affect behaviour and therefore symptomatology.

Consultation: (i) Just about any conversation, (ii) a clinical interview, (iii) a specific kind of conversation in which two or more people explore the nature of a particular problem and the options of how to proceed. The focus does not have to be medical or psychological.

Counter-conditioning: The replacement of one set of conditioned responses by another presented with higher levels of reinforcement (e.g. agoraphobia) with fear of certain situations being replaced by aggressive exposure to such situations to demonstrate that fear is unjustified.

Countertransference: See *Transference*. Countertransference is the analyst's or therapist's corresponding transference onto his or her patient. It would distort treatment, and hence helping the analyst manage countertransference is one of the important aims of a training analysis.

Defences: A range of unconscious psychological mechanisms by which the ego (the sense of integrated self) protects itself from a range of threats which may come from within or from external reality.

Denial: One of the defence mechanisms. For example, pretending to oneself that something very traumatic has not happened, or was not that bad. There are many degrees and kinds of denial, from healthy self-protection through neurosis to some forms of psychosis.

Desensitization: The gradual loss of anxiety/fear following the gradual exposure of a subject to a feared object, usually by ascent of a hierarchy of fear expectations (for example, a person with a phobia of dogs is first presented with photographs of small dogs (such as cairn terriers) and then by photographs of bigger ones, moving on to encountering small and then large dogs in real life).

Dynamic psychotherapy: Psychotherapy that, despite not being classical psychoanalysis, uses theories and principles drawn from psychoanalytic theory.

Evidence-based medicine: This is defined as 'the conscientious, explicit, and judicious use of current best evidence in making decisions about the care of individual patients' (Sackett *et al.*, 1996). All medical practitioners are now exhorted to use this approach. This is perfectly logical; but the practitioner has to be aware that not all patients are the same, and what is sauce for the goose is not necessarily sauce for the gander. If everyone was indeed the same in their responses to treatment, the whole of medical assessment and treatment could be passed over to computers. There is therefore the alternative of *patient-based evidence* in which the experience of one individual (for example, every time that person is ill he responds to treatment X, and even though treatment Y is the recommended treatment for this condition I will still use treatment X) sometimes trumps the requirements of evidence-based medicine.

Extinction (of a conditioned response): Removal of a conditioned response by replacement of reinforcing stimuli or behaviour by different stimuli or behaviour.

Factitious disorder: The intentional creation (feigning) of symptoms of physical or mental disorder for no obvious reason (when it occurs with an obvious purpose it is called *malingering*). This can be difficult to evaluate as such symptoms can also be found in those who have a history of the disorder at other times and are therefore very skilled at simulation (Tyrer *et al.*, 2001).

Flooding: The exposure of a person with a phobia to a feared situation and then preventing escape from the situation so that it is recognized as harmless (compare with *Desensitization* whereby the same result is achieved gradually).

Free association: A term first used by the mathematician and geneticist Francis Galton, who noticed (while travelling about London by public transport) that the movement of one mental phenomenon to another (mental associations) was often not random and could be explained by 'background' or unconscious links that were only possible to identify later by careful analysis. This was taken up by Freud and many others in the development of psychoanalysis as it was viewed as one of the pathways to identifying unconscious wishes.

Generalization: The phenomenon of the extension of one part of learning from a specific situation to a much larger number of (general) situations that share the important part of the original situation.

Insight: This is commonly defined as 'awareness of being ill' in the context of mental illness. So 'insight is maintained' usually is shorthand for saying 'the person recognizes that the experiences he or she is feeling are part of a mental condition rather than objectively real. However, as Anthony David (1990) has emphasized, insight is much more complicated than this and ranges from simple misattribution (e.g. thinking that a voice from the radio is coming from outer space), to cognitive errors (e.g. thinking you are dying from a curse when you are told you have a sexually transmitted disease), systematic biases or idiosyncratic beliefs (including delusions). Almost all people with mental illness have some insight for most of the time. It is also a form of correlation between the patient's beliefs and those of the therapist. Insight is considered lacking if the patient has a different view from the therapist, but of course it may be the therapist that is wrong!

Introjection: The mechanism through which something in the real world 'outside' becomes represented within – for example, when someone gains confidence having done something well, or finds that they take for granted, and as their own, attitudes represented by their culture or sub-culture.

Life events: Events that have the potential for major impact on people's lives and which to some extent are independent of other factors. These can be recorded in terms of their perceived influence, with major events (e.g. the death of child) scoring much higher than others (e.g. moving house in the same town).

Mentalization: This is defined by Bateman and Fonagy (2010) as 'implicitly and explicitly interpreting the actions of oneself and others as meaningful on the basis of intentional mental states', and is particularly used in mentalization-based therapy (MBT) for borderline personality disorder. But it overlaps greatly with mindfulness, one of the key components of dialectical behaviour therapy and mindfulness CBT. I prefer to describe this as 'the capacity for mutual understanding'. If you have the ability to guess correctly at other people's feelings and emotions and can recognise your own then you have good mentalizing abilities.

Nidotherapy: This is a collaborative treatment involving the systematic assessment and modification of the environment to minimize the impact of any form of mental disorder on the individual or on society. It is named after *nidus*, the Latin word for nest, as the nest represents a natural object that will adjust to any shape placed within it. In nidotherapy the person receiving treatment is helped by a therapist (nidotherapist) to change the social and physical environment to make a better fit and thereby revoke the label of mental disorder.

Projection: Seeing an image in the mind (and its attendant feelings) as if it was outside reality. For example, attributing malicious intent to someone when there is no objective reason to believe this.

Psychiatrist: A specialist in mental health who is also a doctor and has a medical degree.

Psychoanalysis: The classical, intensive, long-term psychotherapy developed by Sigmund Freud. It is also applied to the name of the theory on which it is based.

Psychologist: A specialist in the study of the mind. This term includes animal psychologists, specialists in the study of the higher mental functions of other animals, occupational psychologists, specialists in the study of occupational mental functioning, analytical psychologists, who are usually psychotherapists, and clinical psychologists, who have formal training in the practice of psychological assessment and treatment of mental health problems. Chartered psychologists are similar but have a less broad training.

Psychotherapist: Someone trained in one of the many schools of psychotherapy and (ideally) formally recognized as such. A psychotherapist may also be a psychiatrist, a psychologist, or a member of another profession entirely.

Reciprocal inhibition: The term originally used by Joseph Wolpe to describe the phenomenon of desensitization (q.v.).

Schizophrenia: One of the most serious mental illnesses, literally meaning 'shattered mind'; it is characterized by disintegration of mental function with islands of normality linked to major symptoms such as hallucinations (experiencing perceptions such as touch, voices, visions in the absence of any obvious stimulus) and delusions (fixed false beliefs held against all evidence to the contrary).

Systemic theory: Psychological theories (and consequent practice) which emphasize the interactive homeostatic (i.e. self-correcting) processes going on *between* people (e.g. in a group, family or organization) instead of only inside their heads. It represents a psychosocial version of *systems theory* in general which applies to living in natural systems.

Transference: Feelings arising in interrelationships (e.g. in psychotherapy) which the patient attributes to the therapist (for example, feeling generally unliked becomes 'she doesn't like me').

Unconscious (mind): That part of mental functioning of which we are unaware, yet which influences our feelings, attitudes and behaviour. Aspects of the influential unconscious may be 'recovered' in personal reflection, in dreams, in certain experimental situations and in dynamic psychotherapy and psychoanalysis. It is an important but elusive concept. Some theories maintain that the notion of unconscious thinking is a contradiction in terms, if not oxymoronic (mutually contradictive), and that the non-conscious part of the mind is physical rather than psychological. The subject will continue to cause dispute.

REFERENCES

Bateman A, and Fonagy P. (2010). Mentalization based treatment for borderline personality disorder. World Psychiatry, **9**, 11–15.

David, A.S. (1990) Insight and psychosis. *British Journal of Psychiatry*, **156**, 798–808.

Sackett, D.L., Rosenberg, W.M.C., Muir Gray, J.A., Haynes, R.B. and Richardson, W.S. (1996) Evidence based medicine: what it is and what it isn't. *British Medical Journal*, **312**, 71–72.

Tyrer, P., Emmanuel, J., Babidge, N., Yarger, N. and Ranger, M. (2001) Instrumental psychosis: the syndrome of the Good Soldier Svejk. *Journal of the Royal Society of Medicine*, **94**, 22–25. Also reprinted in Czech: Účelová psychóza: syndrom Dobrého vojáka Švejka. *Psychiatrie: casopis pro moderní psychiatrii*, **3**, 151–155.

INDEX

1984 (Orwell), 77

abnormality, concept, 36–7
adaptive functioning, 94
adjustment disorder, 181
Adler, A., 56
aetiology, 155–6
agoraphobia, 82–4, 145, 181
alcohol abuse
   aversion therapy, 91–2
   cognitive-behavioural model, 90
   dialectical behaviour therapy, 92
   social factors, 108
amoeba, 53
analytical psychology, 55
anomie, 104, 181
anorexia nervosa, 60–1
antipsychotics, 31
antiroyalists, 113
antisocial behaviour, 37
anxiety
   cognitive-behaviour therapy, 78
   danger/threat, 110
   life events, 102
   survival, 62
apomorphine, 92
appraisal cognitions, 80
approval, 159
Aquilina, C., 19
archetypes, 55, 56, 181

art therapy, 42, 56, 63–4
arts, 51
astrology, 105
attachment theory, 54, 58–61
auditory hallucinations, 24, 25, 28
authoritarian role, 35, 96
autonomy, 168
aversion therapy, 91–2
avoidance, 75

bad objects, 57
Beck, A.T., 77, 78
behaviour activation therapy, 181
behaviour change, 145–6
behaviour therapists, 42
behaviour therapy, 181
behaviourism, 70–1, 74–7, 182
'being in therapy', 42
beliefs, 89, 90
Bell, Sir C., 12
bereavement, 104, 105
Big Brother, 77
bio-psychosocial model, 5
bipolar affective disorder, 182
   cognitive-behaviour therapy, 78
   manic phase, 36
birth injury, 125
Bloom, H., 54
borderline personality disorder, 64, 158
Bowlby, J., 58

Bradshaw, W., 170
brain
    injury, 125
    scans, 28
    washing, 97, 98
Brasilia, F., 114–15
Bright's disease, 13
Brown, G., 106
Budd, W., 170–1
built environment, 110
Bursten, B., 5

Caplan, G., 167, 168
care
    management, 165
    models, 172–3
case management, 165
cases, 15, 33
cause, 30–2, 155–6
causes, 109–11
chaos theory, 45, 165, 166
charismatic leaders, 62
children
    child psychiatric practice, model of
        teamwork, 162–5
    cognitive-behavioural model, 93
    depression, 163
    play therapy, 64
    superstitions, 79–80
Clark, L.G., 53
classical conditioning, 72–4, 91
classification, 33, 128–34
clinical consultation, 166–7
clinical syndrome, 12–28
clinical trials, 31
cognition, 20
cognitive-behaviour therapists, 42
cognitive-behaviour therapy
    (CBT), 78, 80, 98, 141, 171
cognitive-behavioural model,
    69–100, 124, 125, 139–141, 151,
    158, 161
    applications, 91–3
    behaviourism, 74–7
    central tenets, 79
    cognitive component, 77–9
    criticisms, 93–8
    development, 70–4

differences from other models, 69–70,
    89–91
    guided discovery, 98
    mindfulness CBT, 80
    in practice, 81–8
    relapse, 99
    symptoms, 70
    testing, 79–80
    versatility, 90
cognitive distortions, 77–8
cognitive set, 151
collective unconscious, 55, 182
common-sense, 94
community care, 115
comorbidity, 12
complexes, 47, 182
complexity
    consultative approach, 166–8
    in medicine and psychiatry, 165–6
compulsory admission, 35, 153,
    169–70
compulsory treatment, 35–8, 159
conditioned avoidance response, 76, 84
conditioning, 72
consensus, 127–8
consultation, 166–8, 182
consultative work, 42, 167
consultee, 167–8
consumers, 168
conversion, 32
Cooklin, A., 167
cothymia, 106
counselling, 42, 63
counter-conditioning, 77, 182
countertransference, 48, 182
course of syndrome, 29–30
creative therapies, 42, 64
cultural background, 112, 158

dangerous and severe personality
    disorder, 37
deconstruction, 165
defences, 50–1, 182
delusional mood, 18, 144
delusional perception, 24, 156
delusions, 24, 36, 146
dementia praecox, 107
denial, 51, 182

dependency, 48–9
depression
    children, 163
    cognitive-behaviour therapy, 78
    cognitive distortions, 77–8
    endogenous, 107
    evolutionary adaptation, 62
    hypochondriasis, 84–8
    life events, 106, 107
    loss, 108–10
    neurotic, 107
    reactive, 155
depressive cognition, 89
depressive position, 57
depressive thoughts, 89
deprivation, 108
Descartes, R., 78
descriptive psychopathology, 18
desensitization, 76, 182
development of mental disorders, 147–62
diagnosis, 13, 38, 128–37
Diagnostic and Statistical Manual for
    Mental Disorders (DSM-IV), 128
diagnostic formulation, 18, 21
Dialectical behaviour therapy, 92
disability, 145–6
disease
    definition, 11
    stages of identification, 11–32
disease model, 2, 3, 5, 9–39, 95, 123,
        140–1, 150
    attitudes of doctors, 35
    compulsory treatment, 35–8
    defence of, 38–9
    determining cause and treatment, 30–2
    four tenets, 12
    identification of clinical syndrome,
        12–28
    identification of pathology, 28–9
    natural history (course) of syndrome,
        29–30
    patient as passive recipient of
        treatment, 33–4
    psychoses, 140
    rigidity, 27
    scientific model, 37
    setting boundaries, 32–5
    standard assessment, useful analogy, 19

disintegration, 146–7
dissidents, 113
dissociation, 32
distress, 144
diversity, 175
doctor-patient relationship, 138–9, 157–8
dopamine blockers, 31
drama therapy, 63–4
dreams, 54, 77
drug abuse, 90
drug therapy, 31, 141
Durkheim, E., 104
dynamic psychotherapy, 182

eating disorders
    anorexia nervosa, 60–1
    cognitive-behavioural model, 90
eclectic, 2, 124, 125, 162
ego, 53, 57
Ehrlich, P., 34
Electra complex, 54
electroconvulsive therapy (ECT), 32, 141
electronic circuit concept, 45
Ellis, A., 77
emergent behaviours, 165
emetine, 92
empathy, 158
empowerment, 168
endogenous illness, 107
Engel, G., 5
epigenetics, 29
ethical issues, 146
ethology, 54
evidence-based medicine, 31, 150,
    182–3
evolutionary model, 56, 61–2
examination, 16–7
    mental state, 16–7, 20, 25–6
    physical, 13, 16, 17, 20, 25
experimental science, 70–1, 74
exposure therapy, 76
extinction, 73, 74, 183
Ey, H., 48
Eysenck, H.J., 69, 125

factitious disorder, 28, 183
family history, 19, 22–3
family therapy, 41, 64–5, 118, 164–5

family work, 164, 172
feelings, 45
final common path, 51
first interview, 159
flooding, 76, 183
formalized assessment, 157
free association, 183
Freud, A., 50
Freud, S., 42, 53–4, 170
Freudian slips, 63

gambling, 158
Gaslight (Hamilton), 113–14
'*Gaslight* phenomenon', 114
general systems model, 166
generalization, 75, 183
genetic studies, 30
geological concepts, 45
George III, 30
'giving up', 110
'good enough' parent, 49, 58
good objects, 57
grief, 60, 62, 147
group theory, 64
group therapy, 42, 65
guided discovery, 98

habits, 158, 164
hallucinations, 24, 25, 28, 146
Hamlet, 5, 69
'here and now', 52
hidden depths, 51
hierarchy of models, 148–62
hippocampus, 28
history, 13–6, 19–21, 22–3
hoarding disorder, 141–2
holistic approach, 15
Holmes, J., 61
Holmes, S., 12
Holmes, T.H., 105
home-based care, 172
homosexuality, 97
humanistic psychotherapy, 63
Hunter, R., 16, 35
hydraulic concepts, 45, 96
hydrodynamic concepts, 45
hypochondriasis, 84–8
hysteria, 32, 60

iatrogenic illness, 95
id, 53
ideas of reference, 18, 156
illusions, 146
images, unconscious, 55
imaging, 28
implosion, 76
individual psychology, 56
inferiority complex, 56
informed consent, 6, 168
insight, 145, 183
institutional behaviour, 96
integrative model
    behaviour change, 145–6
    care model, 165
    central tenets, 140
    child and community psychiatric
        practice, 147–62
    complexity, 165–8
    development of mental disorders,
        147–62
    disintegration, 146–7
    distress, 144
    interaction, 137–8
    irrational thinking, 145
    matching to disorder, 140–1
    medical model, 138–40
    patients' views, 168–72
    professional work, 173–4
    resolving conflicts in, 141–3
    symptoms, 144–5
intellectual disability, 93
International Classification of Disease
    (ICD-10), 24, 128–9, 131–6
inter-professional collaboration, 167
inter-professional consultation, 167
interview, 159
introjection, 53, 58, 183
irrational thinking, 145
irritability, 53

James, W., 158
jargon, 18
Jaspers, K., 18
Jung, C.G., 46, 55–6

key workers, 164
Kiosk, Dr, 50

Kipling, R., 41
Klein, M., 57–8

labelling, 111, 136
laboratory tests, 28
Laing, R., 152
language, 52
law, 112
lead, 138
learned helplessness, 96
learning theory, 70, 71–2, 74
letter-writing, 65
levels
    of function, 125, 126
    of illness, 143–7
    matching models, 149–50
life change units (LCU), 105
life events, 105–7, 184
loss, depression, 108–10
lunatic, 105

Macbeth, Lady, 5
'mad', 114, 159
'magic bullet', 34
main complaint, 19, 21–2
maladaptive functioning, 94
mania, 107
marital disorders, 90
McCabe, R., 26
medical model, 5, 138–40
medicalization, 11, 152
memory, 20
mental handicap, 33
mental health consultation, 167
mental health problems, 11
mental illness, 11, 29
mentalization, 61, 184
mental set, 145
mental state examination, 16–7, 20, 25–6
methicillin-resistant *Staphylococcus aureus* (MRSA), 166
Miller, J., 15
Milligan, S., 169
mind, 125
modelling, 83, 95
models
    care, 172–3
    hierarchy, 148–62

interaction, 137–8
matching levels, 149–50
matching to disorder, 140–1
patients' views, 168–72
professional work, 173–4
trouble caused by, 2
moral neutrality, 49
motivation, 97
Mrs Dalloway (Woolf), 170
multidisciplinary teamwork, 35, 127, 141, 162–5, 171, 172
music therapy, 118

narrative therapy, 65
National Institute for Clinical Excellence (NICE), 171
natural history of syndrome, 29–30
negative reinforcement, 73, 74, 92
nerves, 144
neuropsychological tests, 20
neurosis, 50
nidotherapy, 116–17, 141, 143, 184
non-judgmental, 49
non-linearity, 165, 166
non-verbal expression, 52
norms of society, 112
nursing, 173

observation, 12
observer, as part of system, 165
obsessive–compulsive disorder, 98–9
Oedipal complex, 54
open systems, 165
operant conditioning, 72, 74
organizational consultation, 167
organizational hierarchy, 148
organizational psychology, 42
Osmond, H., 5
out-patient care, 172

pain, 53
pan-phobia, 153
panic attacks, 84, 89
paranoid delusions, 22, 24
paranoid position, 57
Parkes, C.M., 60
passivity, 22, 25
pathology, 28–9, 156

patients
  approval, 159
  as consumers, 168
  dependency, 48–9
  empowerment, 168
  informed consent, 6, 168
  involvement in decisions, 6
  as passive recipient of
    treatment, 33–4
  putting in control, 98–100
  viewpoint of models, 168–72
patterns of feelings, 45
Pavlov, I., 70, 72–4
penile plethysmography, 97
personal history, 19, 23
personality disorder, 64, 90, 162
phenomenology, 18
philosophical psychology, 56
phobias, 75–7, 138
  agoraphobia, 82–4, 145, 181
  pan-phobia, 153
  treatment, 76
physical examination, 13, 16, 17, 20, 25
physical treatment, 141
placebos, 15
play therapy, 64
pleasure, 53
Popper, K., 37
porphyria, 30
positive reinforcement, 73, 74
postnatal blues, 144
post-traumatic syndromes, 144
power struggle, 127
predisposition, 155
present condition, history, 20, 24
'pressure cooker' model, 45
prevention, 157–62
previous personality, 20, 23–4
problem-orientation, 135, 136
Procrustes, 126
professional-client relationship, 139
professional work models, 173–4
prognosis, 12
progressive psychotherapy, 63
projection, 48, 184
protectiveness, 49
psyche, 125
psychiatric hospitals, 114

psychiatric nurses, 173
psychiatric team, hierarchy, 35
psychiatrists, 114, 184
psychiatry, 10
  complexity, 165–6
  diagnosis and classification, 128–37
  'soft' branch of medicine, 2–3
psychoanalysis, 42, 184
psychodynamic model, 41–66, 123, 125,
    139–41, 151, 158
  basic principles, 44–52
  Lady Macbeth, 5
  misconceptions, 41
  practical applications, 62–5
  style of clinical thinking, 41
  truth in, 43–4
  variations, 53–8
psychodynamic psychotherapy
  essentials, 52
  supervision, 42
  training, 42
psychodynamic therapists, 42
psychologist, 184
psychoneurosis, 50
psychosis, 140, 146
psychosurgery, 141
psychotherapist, 42, 184
psychotherapy, 141

quantum physics, 45

Rahe, R.H., 105
randomized controlled trials, 31
rational emotive therapy, 77
rationalization, 50
Rayner, R., 74–5
reaction formation, 51
reactive depression, 155
reciprocal inhibition, 76, 184
reframing, 165
rehabilitation, 141
reinforcement, 73, 74
relapse, 99
relationship problems, 145–6
reporting findings, 18–19
repression, 51
residential care, 172, 173
resistant problem, 170–1

rituals, 99
'Room 101', 77
rules of society, 113
ruminations, 99

safety-seeking behaviours, 82
Savage, G., 170
Scadding, J.E., 11, 32
schemas, 95
schizoid personality disorder, 24, 25
schizophrenia, 184–5
    awareness, 26
    brain abnormalities, 31, 161–2
    cognitive-behaviour therapy, 76
    delusional mood, 18, 144
    drug treatment, 31
    identification of clinical
        syndrome, 24, 25
    life events, 107
    natural reaction to oppressive
        conformity, 152
    sluggish, 112–13
schizophrenic spectrum, 22, 62
schizophreniform illnesses, 30
scientific experiment, 70–1, 74
scientist practitioner, 125
scripts, 65
secondary gain, 32
self-feeding, 93
self-harm, 158
self-help, 171–2
Self Help for Your Nerves
    (Weekes), 171
sessional care, 172, 173
Shakespeare, W.
    Hamlet, 69
    Lady Macbeth, 5
shaping, 95
Shaw, B., 73
Sherrington, C., 46
sick role, 95, 157–8
Siegler, N., 5
signs, 12
Simple, P., 50
Skinner, B.F., 70, 74
Skinner box, 74
Slater, E., 9, 39
sleep disorders, 90

sluggish schizophrenia, 112–13
Smith, S., 170
Smith, W., 77
social abnormality, 37
social anxiety, 125–6
social attitudes, 114
social deprivation, 108
social drift, 108
social engineering, 141
social model, 103–19, 124, 125, 140,
    151–2, 158–9
    causes and symptoms of mental
        illness, 109–11
    central tenets, 103
    differences from psychodynamic
        model, 103, 104
    family therapy, 118
    identification of social factors, 108
    music therapy, 118
    nidotherapy, 116–17
    in practice, 108–9
Social Readjustment Rating Scale, 105
social skills training, 139, 141, 173
social workers, 161
society norms/rules, 112–13
somatic delusions, 24
speech analysis, 20
stages, development of mental
    disorders, 147–62
Steinberg, D., 165, 167
stimulus–response link, 72
stories, 65
stress
    'pressure cooker' model, 45
    reactions, 106
suicide
    social factors, 104
    threatened, 85
superego, 53
superstitions, 79–80
supervision, 42
symbolism, 52
symptoms, 144–5
    association with signs, 12
    cognitive-behavioural model, 70
    in different models, 69–70, 96, 140
    social model, 109–11
    substitution, 70, 96–7

syndrome
  identification, 12–28
  natural history, 29–30
systematic desensitization, 76
systemic theory, 64, 185
systems consultation, 167
Szasz, T., 111

Tavistock Institute, 65
teaching, 141, 168
  exercise, 179–80
teamwork. *see* multidisciplinary
  teamwork
Thatcher, M., 63
therapeutic communities, 173
thought disorder, 25, 26
thoughts, 20
training, 42, 141
transcultural psychiatry, 158–9
transference, 48, 185
treatment
  aligned with models, 141
  compulsory, 35–8, 159
  social model, 116–17

triggering events, 155
twin studies, 30

unconscious, 45–7, 185
  collective, 55, 182
  images, 55
USSR, dissidents, 112

van Leeuwen, H., 103
von Economo's disease, 29

Warner, P., 19
Watson, J.B., 70–1, 74–5
Wilson, P., 43
Winnicott, D.W., 49
witch doctors, 111
Wolpe, J., 76
Woolf, V., 170
working hypothesis, 37, 136–7